The Self in Health and Illness

Patients, professionals and narrative identity

Edited by

Frances Rapport

Reader in Qualitative Health Research
School of Medicine
Swansea University

and

Paul Wainwright

Professor of Nursing
Faculty of Health and Social Care Sciences
Kingston University and St George's University of London

Foreword by

Elliot G Mishler

Professor of Social Psychology
Department of Psychiatry
Harvard Medical School

Radcliffe Publishing
Oxford • Seattle

Radcliffe Publishing Ltd
18 Marcham Road
Abingdon
Oxon OX14 1AA
United Kingdom

www.radcliffe-oxford.com
Electronic catalogue and worldwide online ordering facility.

British Library Cataloguing in Publication Data

A catalogue record for this book is available from the British Library.

ISBN-10: 1 84619 112 2
ISBN-13: 978 184619 112 1

Typeset by Lapiz Digital Services, Chennai
Printed and bound by TJ International Ltd, Padstow, Cornwall

Contents

Foreword

O body swayed to music, O brightening glance,
How can we know the dancer from the dance?
                                WB Yeats, *Among School Children*

With surprising speed, the loosely defined field of narrative studies has moved from its early marginal status in the human sciences to a robust legitimacy. Beginning its ascent at some point in the mid-1980s, it now includes a rich, interdisciplinary, still-expanding corpus of theoretical and research studies. Its hallmark is diversity – in theory, method, and subject matter – a feature I have tried to capture by referring to it as a problem-centred area of inquiry. Drawn by its promise to re-humanise the social sciences by throwing off the smothering cloak of positivism, investigators from many disciplines have explored new topics, such as the functions of narratives of resistance by oppressed groups and the narrative structure of legal arguments, and revisited old ones, such as the problem of identity.

The latter has attracted considerable attention, reflecting the substantial body of research focused on life stories, or personal experience narratives. In brief, if you ask people questions about their lives they tell stories that express some version of 'who' they are. There is no tale without a teller, and – as Yeats cautions us in the closing couplet of his poem – we may find it difficult to separate the 'dancer from the dance'. Within the healthcare field, narrative researchers from various health professions and social science disciplines have been particularly interested in the potential impact of disability and illness on patients' identities. The papers assembled together in this book reflect those concerns.

Caught up in the narrative turn at an early point, I welcomed the invitation to write a Foreword as an opportunity to reflect on what we might learn from this collection about current directions in the field. My perspective has been shaped by participation for the past 20 years in an informal, narrative 'interpretive community', the joint product of two interdisciplinary, inter-university groups of narrative researchers who meet regularly to discuss their research. This experience informs my remarks since it has sensitised me both to the diversity of the field and to the importance of a supportive environment that fosters communication among narrative researchers from different disciplines with different approaches.

In their initial call for papers for the special issue of *Medical Humanities* in which most of these papers first appeared, Paul Wainwright and Frances Rapport remark that their interest in the 'nature of the self' was sparked by opposing views of identity expressed by Jerome Bruner, a cognitive/cultural psychologist who has been a strong advocate for narrative studies, and the philosopher, Galen Strawson. They cite Bruner as arguing, in a recent book, that the 'self is a perpetually rewritten story' and that 'we create not just one self-making story but many of them'. The 'job', he asserts is 'to get them all into one identity, and to get them all lined up over time'. Reviewing this book, Strawson not only contests the claim that we 'create' our selves by 'writing' or 'storying' but seems to imply that we may lose our 'selves' that way: 'the more you recall, retell, narrate yourself, the further you risk moving away from accurate self-understanding, from the truth of your being'.

Strawson's view would not spark much interest – or much concern about their work – among narrative researchers. But in addition to their likely general response that identity is expressed and performed through narrative, we find a stronger counter-argument in some of the papers, namely that identities are formed and changed through narratives. For example, Sparkes and Smith argue, in their analysis of types of narrative developed by men with spinal cord injuries, that the creation of new stories of who they are and what they want to do is a 'productive practice' in the development of their new identities. In a similar vein, Roe and Davidson suggest that the process of constructing a succession of increasingly coherent narratives about their experiences, through which they regain ownership of their own stories, is helpful to the recovery process of individuals diagnosed with schizophrenia.

These are strong claims and I highlight them for that reason. They also help sharpen the contrast between different models of the psychological functions of narratives and their related research approaches. In the active or productive model, the focus is on individuals as agents who remake themselves through their stories. In the alternative model of narratives as expressive, that is, as displays of who we are, attention is directed to how stories emerge – and how identities change – within the context of dialogic relationships. Flaming and Kinsella, for example, draw on phenomenology and hermeneutics in exploring how narratives of the self are grounded in relationships and develop and change through time. Having these alternative approaches in the same place is a special bonus since it suggests that the dialectical relation between the productive and expressive functions of narrative deserves more attention in future research.

There is a complex problem of alternative narratives, that is, of stories told about 'what happened' by different actors in the same situation who view it from different perspectives, which is not often addressed in the narrative/identity literature. The importance of such studies is evident in the report by Campbell and Willis of the conflict between physicians and family members about the 'retention' of body organs from patients who have died. This conflict reflects the different and incompatible 'stories' within which they are located. For parents, the person who died was and remains a son or daughter in a still-continuing family story and taking 'pieces' for research or training – particularly without asking for permission – is a violation of the person; for the physician, the liver, heart, or brain is just dead tissue. This analysis adds a new line of theorising to research on competing sociocultural and political meta-narratives, one that opens up relations between structural dimensions of power and collective identities.

The question of multiple or partial identities, alluded to in the earlier quotation from Bruner on our creating many 'self-making' stories surfaces in several papers – Bullington's elderly subjects on their 'aging bodies', Rhys Dent's subject diagnosed with breast cancer trying to manage her twin roles as patient and mother, Mooney's heterosexual man with HIV/AIDS trying to conceal his illness identity. And perhaps as a counterpoint, Rapport's artist maintaining his singular artistic identity and resisting the demands of both the art world and the larger culture, thus, in a sense, making the world around him fit his needs and aims rather than the reverse.

No small collection of papers could represent the full scope and diversity of narrative studies, even within the subfield of patient illness narratives. We would expect to find an emphasis on some issues and trends and a neglect of others, and that expectation is confirmed here. To suggest the distinctive contribution of this particular set of research reports, and to alert readers as to what they will and will not find here, I want to briefly highlight topics that receive special attention.

In addition to the analyses of the productive functions of life stories and of conflicts among narratives from those in different social positions that I referred to earlier, one striking feature of the volume is the emphasis on philosophical approaches to narrative and identity. Three of the papers, one-third of the total – by Bullington, Flaming, and Kinsella – explicitly ground their studies in phenomenology and/or hermeneutics. Bakhtin, Gadamer, Ricoeur are among the principal resources and their models of self, time and narrative are developed into conceptualisations of identity and methods for empirical research. A second theme that receives more than the usual attention in narrative research is the larger sociocultural and political context within which patient narratives are constructed and function, explicitly in Campbell and Willis, Mooney, and Rapport and more indirectly in other papers. Finally, in comparison to much research on personal narratives that relies on one-shot interviews, the studies reported here often involve successive interviews over time with respondents. This allows for charting changes or shifts in identity as expressed in retellings – Mooney, Roe and Davidson, Sparkes and Smith.

In a sense, as is evident from my brief catalogue of the special features of these studies, this is a loose rather than systematic sampling of current work in one sector of the field of narrative studies. Each reader will, I am sure, find some approach or topic missing that she or he believes should have been included. In a sense, this is what marks the field. It is relatively open and fluid, where the motto to let many flowers bloom seems to be the order of the day. Nonetheless, in the end, despite these terms – loose, open, fluid – what we find here is an array of quite systematic approaches to the complexities with which people narrate, perform, and possibly transform their identities through their stories. This is a serious undertaking and the editors and authors of these papers treat it with deep respect for our common struggle to make sense of our lives by achieving identities we can live with.

Afterword

When I began to write this Foreword, I was surprised to find myself referring to the 'interpretive community' of narrative researchers that I have been part of for the past 20 years. At some point, I came to understand why that experience had surfaced. It was a response to my recognition of the fact that the authors of these papers were 'meeting together' for the first time – between the covers of the book. They were not part of a community of researchers sharing ideas, exchanging each others' papers for comments, meeting together to talk about their work. The strength of the collection that comes from its diversity has its downside – there is only one reference in one paper to one of the other authors. Since I believe that each researcher's work can become deeper and more complex through interaction with other researchers from different fields and different perspectives, I have this fantasy that the book might mark the first step in the development of an interpretive community(ies). If this fantasy shades into reality, perhaps each author will read the other papers, email or call his or her colleagues, meet them at their next academic conference, look for friends in their home communities, call a meeting, etc. Try it.

Elliot G Mishler
Department of Psychiatry – CHA
Harvard Medical School
April 2006

Preface

The origins of this book can be traced to a number of chance conversations early in 2004, when one of the Editors (FR) came across a book review in *The Guardian* newspaper.[1] The review was by Galen Strawson, who at the time was Professor of Philosophy at the University of Reading and the review was of a book by Jerome Bruner, *Making Stories: law, literature, life.*[2] As Strawson notes, in his book Bruner claims that the '"self" is a perpetually rewritten story'. He says we are all constantly engaged in 'self-making narrative', in the end becoming 'the autobiographical narratives by which we "tell about" our lives'. Strawson, reviewing the book, took a very different line. Strawson says:

> Every conscious recall brings an alteration, and the implication is plain: the more you recall, retell, narrate yourself, the further you risk moving away from accurate self understanding, from the truth of your being. Sartre is wrong to say that storying oneself is a universal trait, but he's right that it is extremely common, and he is surely right, contrary to the tide of current opinion in the humanities, that the less you do it the better.

We discussed the review between ourselves, considering the differences between Bruner and Strawson and extended the debate to involve other friends and colleagues. If, as Strawson claims, the idea of self as constructed through narrative 'has come to dominate vast regions of the humanities and human sciences – in psychology, anthropology, philosophy, sociology, political theory, literary studies, religious studies, and psychotherapy', the time seemed to us to be ripe for the medical humanities to pay some attention to the problem. Indeed, the division between the technical account of personhood, popular since Locke, and the social construction of self of which Strawson is so critical, might be seen as a kind of paradigm case of the type of problem with which the medical humanities tries to engage. The disagreement between the positions adopted by Bruner and Strawson might be explained, in part, by differences between disciplinary camps. It seems difficult to locate the individual human experience of life, illness and suffering in the taxonomic account of 'self' conceived by the analytic philosophers. Similarly, both the self of the healthcare practitioner and the notion of self that is at stake in dealing with patients, the self of the patient, as understood within the world of the healthcare practitioner, appear to demand a fuller account than they have had in the past. The self is something more than just what John Locke called a 'conscious thinking thing (whatever substance made up of, whether spiritual or material, simple or compounded, it matters not) which is sensible, or conscious of pleasure or pain, capable of happiness or misery, and so is concerned for itself, as far as that consciousness extends'.[3] It seemed to us that the problem was one perhaps requiring an attempt at interdisciplinary working.

We discussed these ideas with Martyn Evans and Jane MacNaughton, the editors of the journal *Medical Humanities*, and they kindly agreed to allow us to edit a special edition of the journal devoted to the problem of the self in health and illness, seeking to combine contributions from academics within and without the field of the medical humanities, from healthcare practitioners from any discipline and from anyone with experience of healthcare. The common concern would be an interest in 'constructions' of narrative selves. We invited people we knew to be interested in the field to write for us and put out a general call for papers, and received an excellent response. The resulting edition of the Journal appeared in December 2005.

The idea of turning these papers into a book was first suggested by Arthur Frank, one of the people with whom we had discussed the original problem. We were delighted when both the editors and the publishers of the journal, the BMJ Publishing Group, agreed to the idea and we have been very grateful for all their support. We hope that republishing the material from the journal in this form will bring it to the attention of an even wider audience.

We are very grateful to Elliot Mishler for his thought-provoking Foreword. Elliot puts his finger on one unavoidable characteristic of a collection of this kind, pointing out that the authors of the chapters 'meet together for the first time' in these pages. Some of our contributors may well know some of the others and we have had the pleasure of meeting most of them. However, Elliot's point is well made: the papers were submitted in response to a Call for Papers, rather than being commissioned as they would have been for the usual kind of edited collection. In Elliot's view this gives the sense that these writers are not part of an existing research community, but offers the intriguing prospect that such a community might emerge and that the contributors might contact each other. We very much hope that this might happen and we will wait with interest to see what might develop if it does.

Paul Wainwright
Frances Rapport
April 2006

References

1 Strawson G (2004) Tales of the unexpected. *The Guardian*, 10 January. http://books.guardian.co.uk/review/story/0,12084,1118942,00.html (accessed 2 June 2006).

2 Bruner J (2002) *Making Stories: law, literature, life*. Harvard University Press, 2002, Cambridge.

3 Locke J (1975) *An Essay Concerning Human Understanding*. Clarendon Press, Oxford.

About the editors and contributors

Editors

Frances Rapport is a social scientist with a background in the Arts. She is Reader in Qualitative Health Research at the School of Medicine, Swansea University, and a Fellow of the Royal Society of Arts. Her research interests include advances in the field of qualitative methodology in healthcare and the social sciences and Assisted Reproductive Technology Medicine. She is currently exploring the scope of using mixed methods and inter-textual data analysis to study general practitioners and psychiatrists' reflections on inhabited workspaces. Recent publications include:

2005 Rapport F, Doel MA, Elwyn G and Greaves D. From manila to monitor: biographies of general practitioner workspaces. *Health: an interdisciplinary journal for the social study of health, illness and medicine.* (In press.)
2005 Rapport F, Wainwright P and Elywn G. Of the edgelands: exploring new qualitative methodologies. *Medical Humanities.* **31**(1): 37–43.
2004 Rapport F (ed). *New Qualitative Methodologies in Health and Social Care Research.* Routledge, London.

f.l.rapport@swan.ac.uk

Paul Wainwright qualified as a nurse in Southampton and had a range of jobs in the NHS before moving into Higher Education. He worked in the Centre for Philosophy and Health Care in Swansea University until 2005, which is where he developed his interest in the Medical Humanities. He is now Professor of Nursing in the Joint Faculty of Health and Social Care Sciences at Kingston University and St George's University of London. His research interests centre around the nature of practices in healthcare, from a philosophical and an empirical perspective. Recent publications include:

2005 Rapport F, Wainwright P and Elywn G. Of the edgelands: exploring new qualitative methodologies. *Medical Humanities.* **31**(1): 37–43.
2004 Wainwright P. The aesthetics of clinical practice. In: M Evans, P Louhiala and R Puustinen (eds) (2004) *Philosophy for Medicine: applications in a clinical context.* Radcliffe Publishing, Oxford.
2004 Pill R, Wainwright P, McNamee M and Pattison S. *Understanding Professions and Professionals in the Context of Values.* In: S Pattison and R Pill (eds) (2004) Values in professional practice: lessons for health, social care and other professions, pp 13–30. Radcliffe Publishing, Oxford.

p.wainwright@hscs.sgul.ac.uk

Contributors

Jennifer Bullington is an Associate Professor and has an academic background in philosophy and psychology as well as a clinical background as a physiotherapist and body-oriented psychotherapist. In 1999 she defended her doctoral dissertation *The Mysterious Life of the Body: A New Look at Psychosomatics* at the Department of Health and Society at the University of Linköping, Sweden. Her main area of research interest is phenomenology and psychosomatic studies. She is a senior lecturer at Ersta Sköndal University College, Department of Health Care Sciences. Recent publications include:

2005　Bullington J, Sjöström-Flanagan C, Nordemar K and Nordemar K. From pain through chaos towards new meaning: two case studies. *The Arts in Psychotherapy.* **32**(14): 261–74.

2003　Bullington J, Nordemar K, Nordemar K and Sjöström-Flanagan C. Meaning out of chaos: a way to understand chronic pain. *Scandinavian Journal of Caring Science.* **17**: 325–31.
　　　 Bullington J. Health as receptivity: a phenomenological interpretation of allostasis. In: IL Nordenfelt and PE Liss (eds). *Dimensions of Health and Health Promotion.* Rodopi, Amsterdam.

jennifer.bullington@telia.com

Alastair V Campbell is Professor Emeritus of Ethics in Medicine in the School of Medicine, University of Bristol and Senior Research Fellow at the Centre for Ethics in Medicine. He is a former President of the International Association of Bioethics. Professor Campbell is a member of the Medical Ethics Committee of the British Medical Association. Until recently, Professor Campbell was Chairman of the Wellcome Trust's Standing Advisory Group on Ethics and Vice-Chairman of the Retained Organs Commission. He is currently Chairman of the UK Biobank's Ethics and Governance Council. Recent publications include:

2005　Campbell A, Gillet G and Jones G. *Medical Ethics* (4e). Oxford University Press, Oxford.

1995　Campbell A. *Health as Liberation.* Pilgrim Press, Cleveland, Ohio.

Alastair.Campbell@bristol.ac.uk

Larry Davidson is Director of the Program on Recovery and Community Health at Yale University, where he is an Associate Professor of Psychology. He is an established investigator who has received national and international recognition for his use of qualitative and narrative methods in conducting research on processes of recovery in serious mental illness, the effectiveness of peer support and consumer-run programmes, and the development and evaluation of innovative recovery-oriented practices and transformation to recovery-oriented systems of care. Recent publications include:

2005　Davidson L, Harding C and Spaniol L. *Recovery from Severe Mental Illnesses: research evidence and implications for practice.* Boston University Center for Psychiatric Rehabilitation, Boston.

2003　Davidson L. *Living Outside Mental Illness: qualitative studies of recovery in schizophrenia.* New York University Press, New York.

larry.davidson@yale.edu

Janet Rhys Dent is a lay member of North Birmingham Medical Research Ethics committee, a writer and creative writing tutor. She has an academic grounding in literature and socioanthroplogy and is particularly interested in the ethical and sociological implications of medical procedures and treatment, narrative ethics and writing for personal development.

The author of articles relating to ethical issues in education and medicine, she is also the author of a forthcoming book, *The Secret History of a Woman Patient* (Radcliffe Publishing, 2007).

janetrhysdent@hotmail.com

Don Flaming is a Nursing Instructor at Medicine Hat College where he teaches courses in nursing research, death and dying, the foundations of nursing, and pathophysiology. He also advises employees of the local health region on how to improve their evidence-based practice. His professional and research interests focus on understanding the educational experience from both the students' and educators' perspectives, especially the role that philosophical insights can play when exploring this phenomenon. Recent publications include:

2004   Flaming D. Nursing theories as nursing ontologies. *Nursing Philosophy.* **5**(3): 224–9.
2003   Flaming D. Orality to literacy: effects on nursing knowledge. *Nursing Outlook.* **51**(5): 233–8.

dflaming@mhc.ab.ca

Elizabeth A Kinsella is an Assistant Professor in the Faculty of Health Sciences at the University of Western Ontario. Anne's interests include: reflective practice, ethical issues in practice, engaging the moral imagination through the arts and health professional education. Her doctoral dissertation examined the philosophical underpinnings of reflective practice, and proposed an elaboration that illuminates the importance of dialogue and discernment. Anne has facilitated numerous workshops on reflective practice across Canada, and published a book entitled *Reflective Practice and Professional Development: strategies for learning through professional experience* (CAOT Publications). Other publications include:

2001   Kinsella EA. Reflections on reflective practice. *The Canadian Journal of Occupational Therapy.* **68**(3): 195–8.

akinsella@uwo.ca

Anabelle Mooney is a Lecturer at Roehampton University in the area of sociolinguistics. Her research interests include the semiotics of law, gender, marginal religious movements and health communication. Her work on HIV has included investigations of quality of life, NGOs and globalisation, particularly in the context of South India. Recent publications include:

2006   Mooney A. Quality of life: questionnaires and questions. *Journal of Health Communication.* (In press.)
2005   Mooney A and Sarangi S. An ecological framing of HIV preventive intervention: a case study of non-government organizational work in the developing world. *Health.* **9**: 275–96.

2005   Mooney A. *The Rhetoric of Religious Cults: terms of use and abuse.* Palgrave Macmillan, Basingstoke.

a.mooney@roehampton.ac.uk

Nigel Rapport is a social anthropologist. He holds the Canada Research Chair in Globalization, Citizenship and Justice at Concordia University of Montreal, where he is Founding Director of the Centre for Cosmopolitan Studies. He is also Professor at the Norwegian University of Science and Technology, Trondheim. His work represents an attempt to understand, as holistically as possible, the complexity of the individual experience of the sociocultural. Most recently he conducted participant-observation fieldwork in a Scottish hospital assuming the role of a hospital porter. Nigel Rapport is author of a number of monographs, including:

2003   Rapport N. *'I am Dynamite': an alternative anthropology of power.* Routledge, London.
2002   Rapport N. *The Trouble with Community: anthropological reflections on movement, identity and collectivity.* Pluto, London.
1995   Rapport N. *Transcendent Individual: towards a literary and liberal anthropology.* Routledge, London.

nrapport@alcor.concordia.ca

David Roe is an Associate Professor at the Department of Psychiatric Rehabilitation at the University of Medicine and Dentistry, New Jersey. His interests lie around recovery from severe mental illness (SMI). He has conducted studies on the ways people with SMI experience themselves in relation to their illness, how these experiences are related to the course of the illness, and the way these emerge through ongoing interactions between person and environment. Dr Roe is also involved in training, implementing and studying Illness Management and Recovery (IMR), an evidence base psychosocial intervention. Recent publications include:

2004   Roe D, Chopra M and Rudnik A. Coping with mental illness: people as active agents interacting with the disorder. *The Journal of Psychiatric Rehabilitation.* **28**(2): 122–8.
2003   Roe D and Kravetz S. Different ways of being aware of and acknowledging a psychiatric disability. A multifunctional narrative approach to insight into mental disorder. *Journal of Nervous and Mental Disease.* **191**(7): 417–24.

droe@ifh.rutgers.edu

Brett M Smith is a Lecturer in Qualitative Research and a member of the Qualitative Research Unit in the School of Sport and Health Sciences at the University of Exeter. His current research focuses on men, sport and spinal cord injury. He is developing work on the lived experiences of becoming disabled through sport and the storied reconstruction of selves; the possibilities of, tensions in, narrative inquiry; and the pull of the body in storytelling. Recent publications include:

2005   Smith B and Sparkes AC. Men, sport, spinal cord injury and narratives of hope. *Social Science & Medicine.* **61**: 1095–105.

2002   Smith B and Sparkes AC. Men, sport, spinal cord injury, and the construction of coherence: narrative practice in action. *Qualitative Research.* **2**(2): 143–71.

b.m.smith@exeter.ac.uk

Andrew C Sparkes is Director of the Qualitative Research Unit in the School of Health and Sport Sciences at Exeter University. Research interests include: performing bodies and identity formation; interrupted body projects and the narrative (re)construction of self; sporting auto/biographies; and the lives of marginalised individuals and groups. He seeks to explore the lived experience of embodiment via multiple forms of representation. Andrew is editor of *Auto/Biography: An International & Interdisciplinary Journal.* Recent publications include:

2005   Sparkes AC, Batey J and Brown D. The muscled self and its aftermath: a life history study of an elite, black, male bodybuilder. *Auto/Biography.* **13**(2): 131–60.
2004   Sparkes AC. Bodies, narratives, selves and autobiography: the example of Lance Armstrong. *Journal of Sport & Social Issues.* **28**(4): 397–428.

sparkes@exeter.ac.uk

Michaela Willis MBE, herself a bereaved parent, has worked extensively with bereaved families over the last 11 years, as a founder member and Chair of the National Committee relating to Organ Retention (NACOR) and the former Chair of the Bristol Heart Children Action Group (BHCAG). The BHCAG was instrumental in obtaining the public inquiry investigating paediatric cardiac services at the Bristol Royal Infirmary. She is now the Chief Executive of the National Bereavement Partnership, a registered charity which she founded in 2003. Michaela holds an MSc in Healthcare Ethics. She served as a Non-Executive Director for the Retained Organs Commission (2001–4) and currently serves as a Non-Executive Director for the Human Tissue Authority (2005), the North Devon Primary Care Trust and is a Council Member of Action Against Medical Accidents (AvMA).

mwillis@natbp.org.uk

Acknowledgements

This book started life as a Special Edition of the journal *Medical Humanities*, published in December 2005. We are indebted to Martyn Evans and Jane MacNaughton, the editors of the journal, for their enthusiasm for the Special Edition and for their patience, encouragement and faith in our work as guest editors. We are also very grateful to BMJ Publishing and in particular would like to thank Karen Taylor, editorial assistant of *Medical Humanities*. Her efficiency and diligence in putting together the special issue led to the smooth running of the publication as did the hard work of Claire Folkes and Ann Lloyd, the BMJ Publishing technical editors of *Medical Humanities*.

A special thank you must go to Elliot Mishler for his continued support and interest in our work. Not only did Elliot present an excellent Masterclass at Swansea University in the field of narratives in health, but his thought-provoking Foreword to the book offers a most fitting lead in to the chapters that follow.

Neither the Journal edition nor this book would have happened but for the efforts of the authors involved. We had an excellent response to our Call for Papers and from the invited authors and are grateful to them all. We would also like to thank friends and colleagues who acted as peer reviewers, for the time and effort involved in considering these works. In alphabetical order these were: Rolf Ahlzen, Ken Boyd, Kate Bullen, Bill Bytheway, Hugh Chadderton, Peter Collins, Lorraine Culley, Ruth Davies, Marcus Doel, Steve Edwards, Richard Evans, David Greaves, Kip Jones, Keith Lloyd, Christopher Maggs, Herman Peininger, Jaynie Rance, Ian Rhys Jones, Gary Rolfe and Brett Smith.

Our thanks must also go to the team at Radcliffe, with a special mention to Gillian Nineham, Editorial Director, for her enthusiastic response and her help and support throughout the process.

We would like to mention our colleagues at Swansea University and Kingston University and St George's University of London who have supported us in our endeavours, in particular Rhys Williams, Keith Lloyd and David Ford at the School of Medicine in Swansea. In addition, Charlotte Thompson and Anouschka Hurley were kind enough to help with typing and collating of some sections of this book.

Finally thanks to family and friends for their belief in our pursuits and their patience!

Introduction: the nature of self and how it is experienced within and beyond the healthcare setting

Paul Wainwright and Frances Rapport

In his recent book *The Healing Tradition*, David Greaves,[1] a former editor of the *Medical Humanities* journal, describes accompanying a hospital consultant on a ward round. He describes how the consultant, having been through the notes, charts, x-rays and lab reports, sat on the edge of the bed, took the patient's hand and asked, 'And how are you feeling in yourself?' To a lay person such a question may be unsurprising. We tend not to describe our feelings in a reductive way, certainly when it comes to illness rather than injury. We may have specific pains in our backs or knees or hips, but we are not usually conscious of pains in the liver or spleen, and even 'stomach ache' is actually a non-specific complaint. And even when we can be more precise we tend, having discussed the specific problem, to move to a more general account. We say things like, 'The trouble is, it (whatever *it* is) makes you feel so rotten', and 'you' here stands for 'yourself' or 'in your self'. As Bruner suggests, '"self" is the common coin of our speech: no conversation goes on long without its being unapologetically used'.[2]

The human body may be reducible to its constituent parts and our ailments may be capable of being described by reference to very few points of data, but indicators such as the partial pressure of oxygen in the blood or the rate of clearance of creatinine by the kidney or the haemoglobin level tell us nothing, necessarily, about how the person feels, in his or her self. Not only do the patient and the clinician tend to have different frames of reference for the experience of illness or disease, the different accounts have different value. Toombs, describing her experience of multiple sclerosis (MS), describes suffering from a particular kind of muscular pain:

> Various tests were performed culminating in a muscle biopsy. The initial pathology report indicated that there was a primary myopathic process going on but there was no explanation as to the cause. Since there was no clearcut definition of the problem, it was also not clear what therapy might be instituted to correct it. I was extremely discouraged by my inability to get around, by the continuing pain, and by the apparent inconclusiveness of the tests. In frustration I commented that, since the biopsy did not indicate what the problem was, nor what to do about it, we seemed to have gained little by performing the procedure. My physician replied, 'Oh but we have! Now we KNOW something is wrong.' For me, as a patient, to know something was 'wrong' was to be acutely aware of my bodily dysfunction and discomfort, and my inability to carry out the most mundane of activities. For the physician, to know that something was 'wrong' was to have 'objective' evidence in the form of an abnormal pathology report with respect to the muscle tissue removed from my thigh.[3]

Thus Toombs *in herself* had known all along that there was something wrong, but it was not sufficient that she felt something wrong *in herself*: medicine required objective evidence of malfunction at the microscopic level.

The body, then, can be reduced to its physical components, to no more than meat, but it is, as Evans memorably suggests, 'meat with a point of view'.[4] The consultant's question, 'How do you feel in yourself?' is inviting the patient to express that point of view, and is inviting the kind of response that may be mediated by or reflect physiological changes – the patient with a low haemoglobin or a high urea level is very likely to feel pretty rotten – but that is not at the level of the biomedical analysis and represents an account that biomedicine may be singularly ill-equipped to accommodate.

The relationship between the self and health and illness seems, on one level, to be almost self-evident. Lance Armstrong describes the day his testicular cancer was diagnosed:

> I questioned everything: my world, my profession, my self. I had left the house an indestructible 25-year-old, bulletproof. Cancer would change everything for me, I realised; it wouldn't just derail my career, it would deprive me of my entire definition of who I was. I had started with nothing... I had become something... Who would I be if I wasn't Lance Armstrong, world-class cyclist?[5]

Our sense of self, of who we are in ourselves and how we feel in ourselves, would seem to be a product of many factors. We can see something of this in the way Armstrong constructs his own identity, his own sense of self. He says:

> I had started with nothing. My mother was a secretary in Plano, Texas, but on my bike, I had become something. When other kids were swimming at the country club, I was biking miles after school, because it was my chance. There were gallons of sweat all over every trophy and dollar I had ever earned...[5]

Armstrong tells us something of his story and at the same time shows us how that story, as it unfolds, defines who he was and is and may become in the future. Some of the events were not of his choosing or under his control, others were, but all contribute to his self, his 'entire definition of who I was'. He starts life 'with nothing' as the son of a secretary from Plano, Texas, and through his aptitude, ability, and extreme effort he becomes 'Lance Armstrong, world-class cyclist' and in the space of a few hours, between driving to the hospital and driving back, he becomes Lance Armstrong, cancer patient, 'a sick person'.

The idea for the themed edition of *Medical Humanities* from which this book developed came in part from a review by Galen Strawson[6] of a book by Jerome Bruner. In his book, *Making Stories: law, literature, life*,[2] Bruner develops the argument that 'we constantly construct and reconstruct our selves to meet the needs of the situations we encounter'.[2] 'Self-making is a narrative art' according to Bruner.[2] Bruner writes:

> A self is probably the most impressive work of art we ever produce, surely the most intricate. For we create not just one self-making story but many of them, rather like TS Eliot's rhyme, 'We prepare a face to

meet/The faces that we meet.' The job is to get them all into one identity, and to get them lined up over time.[2]

But for Strawson this view is anathema. Developing his critique of Bruner and
narrativity he says:

> The further claim is that we create or invent the self specifically by
> 'writing' and 'storying' it. This idea has come to dominate vast regions
> of the humanities and human sciences – in psychology, anthropology,
> philosophy, sociology, political theory, literary studies, religious stud-
> ies, and psychotherapy. Is any of this true? Do we create ourselves? Is
> the narrativity view a profound and universal insight into the human
> condition?[6]

Strawson claims that it is at best a partial truth, and later in the review he com-
plains that:

> Bruner never raises the question of whether there is any sense in
> which one's self-narrative should be accurate or realistic. Those who
> favour the extreme fictionalist or postmodernist version of the narra-
> tive self-creation view don't care about this, both because they don't
> care about truth and because a fiction isn't open to criticism by com-
> parison with reality (it doesn't matter that there is no Middle Earth).
> But honesty and realism about self and past must matter. There are
> innumerable facts about one's character and history that don't depend
> on one's inventions. One can't found a good life on falsehood.[6]

Leaving aside questions of what is meant by 'accurate or realistic', it seems that
Strawson is taking the narrative construction of self, Bruner's 'storying', as no
different from fiction, as if a story is inevitably or almost always a fiction.
Armstrong's story and the self that emerges from that story do not 'depend on
[his] inventions' and in agreeing that Armstrong himself is a 'work of art', a self-
made and perpetually rewritten story, we are in no sense committed to the
assumption that this is a life founded on a deliberate falsehood.

   In philosophy the self is a contested notion and we have no intention of
attempting to settle the contest here. Strawson himself presents self-experience
as fundamental to human life, and defines it thus:

> By 'Self-experience', then, I mean the experience that people have of
> themselves as being, specifically, a mental presence; a mental some-
> one; a single mental something or other. Such Self-experience comes
> to every normal human being, in some form, in early childhood. The
> realisation of the fact that one's thoughts are unobservable by others,
> the experience of the sense in which one is alone in one's head or
> mind, the mere awareness of oneself as thinking: these are among the
> very deepest facts about the character of human life.[7]

It is difficult to see how we are to make sense of self-experience and the deep-
est facts about the character of human life other than in the context of the
narrative within which that life is embedded. We may be able to make neutral,
generalisable ontological statements about some abstract notion of the self as a
kind of thing, 'a kind of bare locus of consciousness, void of personality, but still

for all that a mental subject'.[7] However, in the context of healthcare practice, for example, one would want to include three other characteristics of the self that Strawson also discusses, but dismisses as unnecessary – the self as:

* a *persisting* thing, a thing that continues to exist across hiatuses in experience
* an *agent*
* something that has a certain character or *personality*.

Strawson argues that a minimal set of characteristics of the self does not need to include these three. In everyday life, however, we tend not to experience ourselves or the selves of others, Zen-like, as bare loci of consciousness, 'void of personality'. Human interaction is intimately bound up with these very characteristics, and any attempt to understand our selves and others, as people, as patients or as healthcare professionals, in varying forms or relations to each other, must necessarily take into account the unique particularity of the self and its story.

The chapters in this book, from a variety of perspectives, address the problem of self as experienced within and beyond the healthcare setting, offering commentaries on how the self can be constructed, whilst illuminating the unique selves of the writers. We open with a chapter by Nigel Rapport, who considers the life of the painter Stanley Spencer in terms of self-artistry and the projected self. Concentrating on 'the existential power of individuals to create and lead their own lives', Rapport describes Spencer's ability to construct a social environment, through creative output, that is created predominantly in his own image. Striving to be his own man, suggests Rapport, is both 'life creating' and enhancing of others' lives. Elizabeth Kinsella offers a general overview of how the self is constructed through three perspectives – the unitary, the fragmented and the dialogical. Kinsella encourages us to examine ethical relationships and the inter-subjectivities that come to light when we engage with others, reflected in the inter-subjective practices of healthcare professionals. These first two papers lay the grounds for three broad themes: a) constructions of self through the body, b) constructions of self through the mind, and c) patients, professionals and sense of self.

The self as embodied is explored in the writings of: Anabelle Mooney (HIV narratives), Andrew Sparkes, Brett Smith (elite sport and the traumatised body), and Jennifer Bullington (the aging body). Mooney views the body as the essential property of our existence, defined in both its explicit and implicit aspects. She describes her HIV-positive respondent's inward and outward portrayals of a stigmatised existence, concluding that our inward mechanisms of storytelling are often surmised rather than explicit in our stories. Mooney reveals the feared and unspoken aspects of illness narrative, suggesting that 'what is feared is the way in which others will write his illness on his body', and offers insights into the spoken and unspoken understandings we give to health and illness. Sparkes and Smith develop ideas surrounding the embodied self through analysis of interviews with sportsmen disabled by spinal cord injury. Using the concepts of metaphor, notions of time and different kinds of hope, as well as the application of Frank's chaos, quest and restitution narratives, Sparkes and Smith argue that experience is shaped by the lives we lead, represented by spoken narratives that convey 'the profundity of human experience'. Bullington describes a phenomenological study of the aging body and its influence on sense of self and identity. Bullington remarks that aging does not necessarily result in negative experiences of self and is revealed through three very different typologies: 'existential awakening' – reorienting one's priorities in life; 'making it good enough' – battling against the aging body; and 'new possibilities' – accepting the aging process.

The relationship between mental illness and the construction or maintenance of self are explored by David Roe and Larry Davidson, who consider the experience of schizophrenia, disruption to selfhood, and the recreation of the life story through recovery from illness. Roe and Davidson suggest that re-authoring of life is an integral process towards illness recovery and although life events can be fragmented for the person suffering from schizophrenia, a strong sense of self can be recovered in time.

Two chapters on the role of patients and professionals from the medical and lay perspectives come from Janet Rhys Dent and Don Flaming. Rhys Dent explores the conflict between motherhood and patienthood, describing her personal journey through breast cancer and arguing that our many identities are shaped by ethical questions of how to lead a good life. She examines her own illness and the 'richness of individual selfhood'. Don Flaming moves from the patient to the professional agenda when he examines the experience of becoming a professional nurse. Flaming applies Ricoeur's understanding of narrative and *mimesis* to offer a reflexive presentation of 10 student nurses' experiences. Flaming discusses continuity of experience from past through present to anticipated future and considers the self to be 'made up of a mixture of past identities that play an integral role in present understanding and experience'. The last chapter is by Alastair Campbell and Michaela Willis, reflecting on professional and patient orientations to self and the difference between medical and lay positions. Taking the example of the post-mortem retention of children's organs, Campbell and Willis suggest that different discourses serve different purposes in the health and illness arena. Medical discourse is a functional discourse pertaining to scientific goals, whist lay understanding is based on shared human experience and the embodied self.

These chapters come together through their use of constructions of self in health and illness narratives in their vision of the self as repairable through the telling and retelling of the story. Central to all these accounts is the importance of the 'point of view' of the person whose self is at stake. This is not about Strawson's bare loci of consciousness, 'void of personality'. It is, rather, about the interaction between our interests, our preferences and our relationship with and responses to the events in our lives. The authors in this issue concentrate on self-control and self-determination, though they may differ in their responses to the ability of individuals to 'write' their own narratives. Rapport, for example, argues for 'the existential power of individuals to create and lead their own lives', whilst Campbell and Willis point to 'a gulf between medical and lay understandings of the human body and its relationship with the human person'. The writers grapple with the relationship between body, mind and self and much time is spent deliberating on the embodied nature of self. Authors question whether the body is quintessentially linked to a sense of self and selfhood: as Mooney suggests, as humans we are embodied but we are not reducible to our bodies. However, Mooney goes on to reflect that our bodies are an 'essential property of our existence'. The authors of these chapters frequently adopt an emotive and reflexive style. In Rhys Dent's illness memoir, for example, self-reflection plays a major role in the story, as she argues that 'the reflexive process is part of this state of being'. Bullington and Flaming, on the other hand, both use reportage to convey the words and feelings of others and there are many examples of emotive writing styles as writers consider the narratives of their study participants. Sparkes and Smith concentrate on the mood of the participants they interviewed: 'In chaos Jamie feels swept along, without control, by life's fundamental contingency' and Mooney, in an attempt to stay true to her participant's presentation, comments: 'I quote John at length in an attempt to give voice to his story.'

This body of work would seem to support Bruner's claim that 'there is no such thing as an intuitively obvious and essential self to know, one that just sits there ready to be portrayed in words'. He goes on: 'Self-making is, after all, our principle means for establishing our uniqueness, and a moment's thought makes plain that we distinguish ourselves from others by comparing our accounts of ourselves with the accounts that others give us of themselves.'[2]

If we accept this view of the self as constructed, we must also be aware of the impact of the events in our lives that shape the selves that we are and that we become. My self as healthcare professional, as academic and as patient co-exist together and alongside the many other facets of my self. The chapters in this book offer rare insight into the nature of the self and its construction.

References

1 Greaves D (2004) *The Healing Tradition: reviving the soul of Western medicine*. Radcliffe Publishing, Oxford.
2 Bruner J (2002) *Making Stories: law, literature, life*. Farrar, New York.
3 Toombs SK (1993) *The Meaning of Illness: a phenomenological account of the different perspectives of physician and patient*. Kluwer, London.
4 Evans M (2002) Reflections on the humanities in medical education. *Med Educ*. **36**: 508–13.
5 Armstrong L (2001) *It's Not About The Bike: my journey back to life*. Yellow Jersey Press, London.
6 Strawson G (2005) Book review: tales of the unexpected. http://books.guardian.co.uk/review/story/0,12084,1118942,00.html (Accessed 11 October 2005.)
7 Strawson G (1999) The self and the SESMET. *Journal of Consciousness Studies*. **6**: 99–135.

Chapter 1

The power of the projected self: a case study in self-artistry

Nigel Rapport

This chapter concerns power, but not power as conventionally understood and represented in social science. Rather than an appreciation of the structural power of what is institutional, collective, impersonal and not individual to create and/or curb what is individual, this is an essay concerning the existential power of individuals to create and lead their own lives.

More precisely, the issue which the chapter sets out to examine is the relationship between consciousness and control: between consciousness of an idea of self in the world, and control over one's individual life in the world. Insofar as persons lead their lives in terms of objectives and criteria of evaluation which are of their own formulation and deployment, do they thus put themselves in positions to ameliorate or even escape the influence of social conditions, factors and forces beyond themselves? If we treat their lives as their own 'life projects', their actions can be seen to be answerable, largely or wholly, to their own worldviews and the conscious fulfilment of these, and not to ideologies, social structures and the structures of the unconscious and embodiment, the so-called prison houses of language and history. Self-consciousness – the exercise of a certain 'self-intensity', projecting one's self along a determined life course – equates with a freedom from the conditions of external circumstance beyond the self.

I explore this issue by bringing together social/scientific and aesthetic analysis[1] in an examination of the life and work of one particular individual: the English painter Stanley Spencer (1891–1959). In constructing an artistic oeuvre of great originality and vision, Stanley Spencer, I shall argue, exhibited a large degree of singlemindedness in his life – singlemindedly focused on a certain life project – and thereby achieved a remarkable order and control in and over the course of his life and the things to which he consciously attended while living it. He succeeded in placing himself in the middle of an abundantly meaningful and intense life narrative; this did not entail subordinating his life to his art so much as intending to live his life as an artwork, as a manifestation of his artistic vision.

Here is how Stanley Spencer is introduced by his first biographer, Maurice Collis:

> He stands a giant (though physically he was a very small man) who was never deflected from his main concern, which was to express himself. His story is bound up with three women in particular [Hilda Carline, Patricia Preece and Daphne Charlton], and also a fourth [Charlotte Murray]. He was influenced by them for a time, but remained unchanged in essentials. They people his art from 1927 till his death and are a recurring subject of his writings. But he was a

recluse at heart, a paradox of which his [posthumous] papers leave no doubt.[2]

The question I pose is whether Spencer's construction of a beautiful, involved and extensive worldview translates into his being able to be described as having control over his life. What is the relationship between the edifice, the narrative, the 'work of art' which Spencer created in and as his life, and his influence over those forces and those others which might otherwise claim a hold over his life? While I do not directly address the question of happiness, of whether his pursuit of a life project was responsible for Stanley Spencer (or those around him) being happy or unhappy, an issue of wellbeing does become relevant. I explore the extent to which Spencer's self-intensity and self-artistry gave rise to a kind of fitness or strength: of character, of identity. Consciousness of an idea of self in the world, and living to project that idea in action, may be instrumental in effecting a kind of ontological wellbeing.

Before we meet Spencer in more detail, I introduce some concepts and terms that aid the analysis.

'Displacement'

My point of analytical departure is the concept of displacement. Etymologically, the word derives from Old French: a negation of place. 'To displace' is to shift or remove or oust from an erstwhile proper, usual, official or dignified position or place, while 'displacement' is a measure of difference between an initial and a subsequent position and embodies movement (*Shorter Oxford English Dictionary*). Hence, a 'displaced person' is a refugee or stateless person, someone removed from his country as a prisoner or slave (*Chambers Twentieth Century Dictionary*).

However, a negation of place, an overcoming of place, might also be conceived of as a positive move, and displacement as a conscious and creative act by which an individual shifts and removes and ousts himself or herself (and perhaps others) as a route to growth. Displacement affords a distance, and a measurement of difference, between an initial identity and a subsequent one. Becoming a refugee or exile from a social milieu or relationship or lifeworld, becoming someone else, the individual assures himself or herself of a vantage point from which to look sideways at their life and consciously create anew. 'Power', as the early American 'transcendentalist' philosopher, Ralph Waldo Emerson, proposed, 'resides in the moment of transition from a past to a new state, in the shooting of the gulf, the darting to an aim'; while it 'ceases in the instant of repose'.[3]

In displacement lies a source of personal, 'existential' power to be and to do.

I am encouraged in this view by the thoughts of the contemporary Emerson scholar, George Kateb. To stay in one place (intellectually or emotionally), Kateb asserts,[4] is to put at risk one's capacity for experience and creativity. Indeed, even to come to know oneself it is necessary to some degree to become alienated or estranged, and thus to see oneself as from a distance; one explores and becomes oneself. Displacement thus encourages what Emerson called 'self-reliance'. Periodically examining oneself and thinking through one's own thoughts, one is not the self same person as the non-displaced one. Moreover, the self one becomes is not constructed merely out of the givens of social milieux and historical circumstance. Displacement has shifted, in an idiosyncratic way, the context of that life: the criteria of judgement upon which it might rely. Displacement gives rise to a habit of self-judgement and self-authentication, the life becoming answerable to questions posed of it by its individual owner, not (or not only) its consociates in its social milieu. The life becomes a self-narrated one.

Kateb calls such a process one of self-recovery: it is an arriving 'home', coming to live 'in one's own place'.[4,5] It is the case, moreover, that the displaced and self-examined person is better able, possibly, to withstand (deny, escape) the constructions made of him or her by others, and the categorising. A sense of the course, the trajectory, of one's own life, knowing where one has moved from and could be moving towards, affords one distance from the placements of others.

'Existential power' and 'in order to' motives

Emerson's statement concerning the power of movement and becoming which I quoted above ends as follows:

> This one fact the world hates; that the soul becomes; for that forever degrades the past, turns all riches to poverty, all reputation to a shame.[3]

On the question of displacement, certainly, analysts from Marx and Durkheim, through Freud to Heidegger and Homi Bhabha, would degrade the notion by identifying it with alienation and anomie, homelessness and exile: with individual powerlessness and lack or loss of control. Analysts fight shy of welcoming the radical newness of the displaced 'soul', the unpredictability and non-classifiability to which its idiosyncratic 'becoming' might be party.

This also accords with a more general social scientific tendency to regard the individual actor as 'put upon' rather than 'putting on', not so much 'self-motivated' as 'socially driven'.[6] Identity becomes wholly a matter of social relations, of what particular social settings cause, construct, classify, elicit. Phenomena such as displacement then become attributes of social milieux, of their conditions and relations, rather than aspects of life which an individual person might be consciously and creatively responsible for effecting. In Alfred Schuetz's designation,[7] causal or 'because' motives predominate in conventional analytical treatments of behaviour in social milieux, while intentional or 'in order to' motives rarely figure beyond the realm of pathology. In the rush to deconstruct the 'political power' of techniques of influence and oppression, a recognition of the 'existential power' to act and constitute identity is lost.[8] That is, a focus on 'institutional processes of governance' eschews a broader conceptualisation of 'the power to do, the capacity to achieve things or projects'.[9]

Questions such as how individuals cope with life or find meaning in the face of suffering or change become overdetermined by questions of social domination, hierarchy, and control.

I would wish to turn this around, however, and, as with the according of a positive characterisation to displacement (regarded as a source of personal power), locate forces of behavioural determination, of the instituting of meaningful worlds, in the individual as such. I would go so far as to say that there are only 'in order to' motives; 'because' motives are what we formulate out of bad faith in order to claim that something or someone other than ourselves is responsible for what we feel, think, say or intend. 'Bad faith' is a Sartrean notion,[10] and existentialism is the moral philosophy that has most determinedly, perhaps, argued the case I would substantiate in this chapter.[11] Individual consciousness creates the meaning of the world and the objects in it, the existentialist claims, rather than that consciousness being the internal manifestation of another, extraneous force – such as Society, the Unconscious or God. We have a freedom to shape our own individual destinies. Awareness of this, however, can cause anguish; we are fearful and unconfident concerning the consequences of our action or our inaction, and our responsibility concerning the choices and decisions of our lives. Hence our flight into 'inauthentic living' and lies. Confronting our authentic selves in their aloneness is frightening and so we shirk the responsibility, in bad faith, and say our choices, our lives, are determined: by our religious doctrines, our personal pasts, our cultural traditions. For our freedom in a fluxional universe we substitute orderly systems, theoretical schemas and determinate structures. This is both a trick which we play on ourselves and on others, and which others would play on us; it is a means of control. Impersonal and extraneous 'because' motives serve the interests of those who would exercise power over others.

It is the case, however, that (to adapt a phrasing of Alfred Whitehead's) such impersonal idioms usher in a 'fallacy of misplaced concreteness' concerning the order of the world and its source: the ideological and merely conventional are taken and mistaken for the real.

'Genius' Nietzsche wanted to prescribe as something to be acquired, something one grew into.[12] My emphasis here, too, is on the developmental aspects of self-intensity or singlemindedness: they are matters of positive feedback. The practice of living 'in order to', of framing one's life in terms of a life project, bestows certain qualities of character on its exponents. Indeed, having and maintaining a life project, expecting to see projects of displacement, change and growth through to completion, may be found to be the most important element in the life project's effectiveness. As in a dialectic, the individual practising of a life project may be responsible for the continuing disposition to keep on practising: practice itself may be the key to the power accrued to control the trajectory of the life imbued by a life project.

Stanley Spencer and the metaphysics of love

Let me illuminate this thesis by turning the attention of the chapter to one life in particular, that of Stanley Spencer: to his imaginative, painted displacements, and their effects on his life. I begin with two quotations:

> I have always looked forward to seeing what I could fish out of myself. I am a treasure island seeker and the island is myself.[2]

> Being with Stanley is like being with a holy person, one who perceives…he is the thing so many strive for and he has only to be. […] Stanley's home seems to be the whole world.

> Hilda Spencer[13]

In his biography of Stanley Spencer, Kenneth Pople[13] offers an interpretation of Spencer's early pen and ink sketch, *The Fairy on the Waterlily Leaf*.

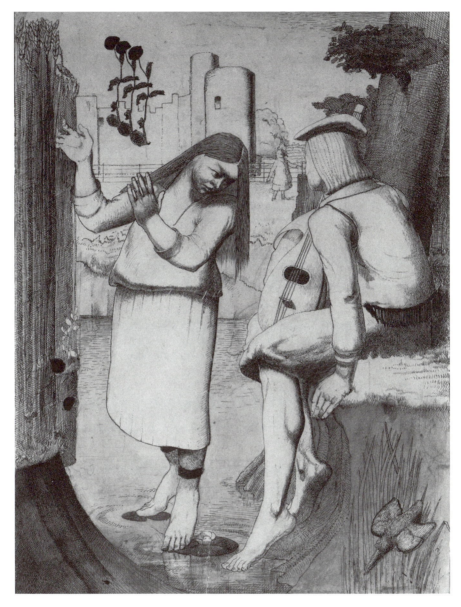

Figure 1.1 *The Fairy on the Waterlily Leaf*, Stanley Spencer, 1910 (41.9 x 30.5 cms).
Copyright: Estate of Stanley Spencer/SODART 2006. All rights reserved (DACS).
Source: Stanley Spencer Gallery, Cookham, Berks., UK/Bridgeman Art Gallery.

The sketch was drawn in 1910 when Spencer was 19, at the request of a Miss White, to illustrate a fairy story she had written. She was not pleased with the result, however, and rejected it. Spencer was puzzled by the rejection and disappointed. Nine years later he again gave it as a gift, this time to his friend Ruth Lowy and her betrothed, Victor Gollancz (the publisher), and again was asked what it meant. He replied that it was a fairy on a water lily leaf but that beyond that he did not honestly know what the picture was all about. 'I was loving something desperately,' Spencer later wrote of this time, 'but what this was I had not the least idea.' What this something was, Pople suggests,[13] was Spencer's dawning awareness of the miracle of love as such: Spencer's 'metaphysic of love' as it was to become. Drawn from deep personal feelings as yet unclarified, it is this that the sketch sets out to honour.

Pople elaborates as follows.[13]

Spencer's fairy, no elfin, is a sturdy girl seemingly impossibly posed on two water lily leaves above a pond. She is being courted by a prince in Renaissance dress (in the form of a certain youth, Edmunds, a male model from Spencer's life class at the Slade School of Art, London). The fairy figure is a representation of the village girl Dorothy Wooster, with whom Spencer had been a school pupil at Cookham-on-Thames. In order to imagine a prince's love for a fairy – the theme of Miss White's original story – Spencer has assembled images from his own experience; in this way he sought to reproduce the emotion of the theme. He draws Dorothy, therefore, beautiful and impossibly buoyant (physically) because he has loved her (metaphysically): the reality of the imagery becomes subservient to the emotion he feels for what is imaged. As for the water, he chose a little sandy beach by the bank of the Thames which he knew from happily playing there as a boy. Finally, he adds scale to the central scenario by diminishing Dorothy's size relative to a row of wheat stalks on her right, and he adds perspective by way of three flowers or marsh plants which he draws in the top left-hand corner. From one perspective the plants seem to have been thrown up into the air by a juggling Dorothy (one of Spencer's elder brothers became a professional juggler). But from another perspective, the marsh plants suggest that Spencer wishes us, like the prince, to be looking down on the scene as from above: to see the artist as having made the vertical height of the sketch into a horizontal expanse of clear water. We and the prince are looking through the water of the pond at the fairy as through a plate-glass window.

The fairy's world is enchanting and lovable but also enchanted and intangible – as enchanted perhaps as the world Spencer hears through music (thus the crotchet-like shape of the plants), and as intangible as his (dawning) world of love still is for him. The fairy is an emanation of that world, but she must return there when the music stops; the prince cannot follow (any more than Spencer could follow the village girls into their world or find his visions in their disappointing conversation).

Nevertheless, in the picture there is the hint of love transcending the boundaries between worlds and their displacements: the physical and the spiritual, the everyday and the heavenly. Also in the picture are the elements of a visionary world which brings together Spencer's local experience and his dreams and hopes of redemption through love, themes which were significantly to characterise his mature art. Manifesting a 'metaphysic of love' was, indeed, to become his life project.

An artful autobiography

In 1938 some friends (including Victor Gollancz) tried to encourage Spencer to write his autobiography; it would help him explain himself to a public becoming distanced by (what John Berger would dub) the intrinsic 'oddness' of his paintings' personal iconography.[14] At first Spencer was quite taken with the idea, for in writing an autobiography he would be seeing his life as a whole, and the 'constant something in myself that I consider to be the essential me that I like'. He would compose not a linear chronological narrative but, as it were, a stroll through his life, with digressions and pauses as the mood took him, and in different genres and styles; chronological development was less important to account for than sentimental.

Eventually, however, Spencer decided against it; if people would not understand his paintings, then why should they understand his explanations? Nonetheless, he did begin to write in private. For the next 21 years he composed diaries, journals, random jottings, extensive essays and unsent letters.[15] He wrote obsessively and kept every scrap: entreaties, memories, fantasies, philosophies, lovemakings; about and to his paintings, wives, family, friends and himself. Collected in trunks, he would dip into the storehouse, the treasure chest, to reread, reannotate, repaginate and rearrange; the writing, he explained, meant he could sort out his thoughts. (Archives are today housed at the Stanley Spencer Gallery, Cookham, and the Tate, London.) In seeking a fuller appreciation of Spencer's art, then, the displacements he achieved through it, and the place of both the art and the displacements in the conscious control he exercised over his life, it is apposite to borrow a selection of Spencer's words as accompaniment and counterpoint.

Spencer's art, I want to argue, was something he used both to prescribe a general metaphysic for earthly life and to describe – reflect, correct and redeem – his own life in particular. It amounted to a life project through which he succeeded in living on his own terms.

Spencer surprised people because, when asked if he believed in God, he never knew what to say. Certainly he cherished no notions of an intimate figure, and he was appalled by those who made religion an excuse for dividing believers from non-believers, members from non-members, and instituting a certain discipline on the world and its beings:

> It is for me to go where the spirit moves me, and not to attempt to ally
> it to some known and specified religion.[13]

Nevertheless, a good place to start the story of Spencer's art is with his Wesleyan Methodist upbringing. This, together with Gladstonean liberalism, permeated his childhood. Here was a value placed on non-monetary things and a faith in perfect universal love, mediated by a one-to-one relationship with God which was attainable on earth. All came together in the imagery of the Bible and services in Cookham Wesleyan chapel: homely, gentle, secure, comfortable and productive. It gave onto a coherent world order whereby, to an imaginative boy and youth, Cookham village seemed to manifest a 'sacred presence'. Here, the natural and the supernatural commingled and visions might be taken for granted. If the family home was the major part of the terrestrial world, then maids talking to themselves in the attic were likely communing with angels: the biblical shepherds watched their flocks on the field below Cliveden Woods, and Cookham churchyard was the path to Eden. The eternal stories of the Bible Spencer located in his own parochial childhood environment, translating their drama and fiction into the reality of his own familiar, everyday experiences:

> I became aware that everywhere was full of special meaning and this
> made everything holy... I saw many burning bushes in Cookham.

I observed this sacred quality in most unexpected quarters. [Cookham]:
holy suburb of heaven.[15]

Cookham simultaneously inspired Spencer and grounded him: allowed him to see
universal truths and provided him with contact with and bearings to the here and
now. The sense of the village representing an earthly paradise stayed with him
throughout his early adulthood. The experience of London and the Slade (then
under the influence of continental art movements such as Post-Impressionism,
Cubism, Vorticism and Expressionism) only made him more sure: everything in
Cookham was cosily innocent and of the morning. Sitting in the family pew at
church one morning in 1915, hearing the activities of the village and the river
going on outside, and again having the sense of the holiness, the sanctity, of the
whole – church and village, 'sacred' and 'profane' – Spencer explains how he had
the idea of taking his 'in church' feeling 'out of church' in his art, transferring an
act of worship to seemingly secular rituals, people and places:

> The thing which interests me and always has done is the way that
> ordinary experiences or happenings in life are continually developing
> and bringing to light all sorts of artistic discoveries.[16]

It was an idea (a unity and a stillness) that would initially be disrupted by the
war, but to which he would return thereafter with redoubled inspiration and
zeal. To an extent, his experiences in the First World War provided a decisive
rupture to Spencer's life and the innocence of his vision. Thereafter, 'Cookham'
represented a rapturous golden age he must now be intent on recapturing: inter-
vening experiences had to be redeemed.

As a medical orderly and latterly a soldier, he had succeeded in mentally escap-
ing a detestable deindividuation and regimentation, finding a personal spirituality
in menial tasks and everyday routines (courtesy of Augustine's *Confessions*), but it
was not until he began painting again that a full catharsis was achievable:

> The first place an artist should find himself is in prison. The moment
> he realises he is a prisoner, he is an artist, and the moment he is an
> artist, he starts to free himself. [Painting] redeemed my experience
> from what it was; namely something alien to me. By this means I
> recover my lost self.[15]

Marrying his thoughts and feelings to people, places and events around the
village – the divinity of their occupations, the ritual of their daily activities – was
to create something holy.

The war was not, however, the only disruption of a major, even tragic, kind in
Spencer's life. His discovery of sex; his marriage to fellow artist Hilda Carline
(1925); his polygamous desire for Patricia Preece; his divorce from Hilda (1937);
his estrangement and divorce from Patricia; his feelings of terrible loss over Hilda;
his persecution by a censorious public; his relative poverty; and his peripatetic
existence (moving between houses at Cookham, Bourne End, Durweston, Steep,
Petersfield, Hampstead, Poole, Burghclere, St Ives, Swiss Cottage, Leonard
Stanley, Port Glasgow and Epsom) – all of these precipitated crises of consciousness. In each instance, however, it was in his artworld (his writing as well as his
painting) that Spencer successfully found equilibrium: a continuity and coherence to the narrative of his life, redemption for what had passed, joy in what was

now, and hope for what was to come. Above all, art provided a fulfilment which was missing in life; art created order out of the disruption, the chaos, of life:

> I am aware that all sorts of parts of me are lying about waiting to join me. It is the way I complete and fulfil myself.[14]

There is, however, more. To this personally cathartic displacement he will marry a supernatural (initially Wesleyan but increasingly pantheistic, even Buddhist) iconography. Heaven and earth are innocently unified, as are races, nations and creeds, men and women, humans and animals, self and other, secular and numinous, bodily and spiritual desire, innocence and experience. While Spencer rejected the liturgical literalness of canonical religion, he still employed the paradigm of Christianity as a resource because it offered a sense and interpretation (one among many possible ones) of the disparate mysteries of the world – and the wonder of experiencing it. What Spencer asked of his audience was not necessarily empathy, nor even sympathy, with his personal vision and representation of this universal consciousness, but an acknowledgement that existence is something whose awesomeness they sensed too. Ultimately, Spencer's vision was also a parochial one: a cult of the sacred self which focused not on Jerusalem, or Paris or Rome, but on the provincial world of Cookham. If the Christian Bible was an allegory of a great truth about the world, then Cookham was too, if its 'pages' were read with the vision that Spencer's art would provide; happenings in Cookham represented a pageant of revelations equivalent to those in the Bible, and Spencer's destiny was to relate the wonder and awe of the one to the other.

It was as if people and events in Cookham were communicants of a church of which he was the priest. Here was a deeper level of human and spiritual consciousness which brought about a new, true state of being, a more magnificent and beautiful way of life, which he saw 'out of doors' in Cookham. Like a mediaeval artist/craftsman/villager, Spencer would endeavour to capture the essence of these manifestations of ordinary local life for local people. For in the same way that Cookham was imbued with a divine truth, so too was he, Spencer. The apparent unchangingness of Cookham revealed an everlasting, mysterious rhythm: the recreation of life from death; the emergence of form from meaningless chaos. Likewise, from the random pieces which the world of the senses continually emptied into his brain, he would create art and reveal the wonder of the identity of each thing on earth, and hopefully transmit something of the ecstasy that this led him to feel:

> [A mass of] inward, surging meaning, a kind of joy, that I longed to get closer to and understand and in some way fulfil.[17]

His vision afforded Spencer a form of transcendence.

Finally, through his art, Spencer would not only celebrate his existence (its conflicts, disorders, and discords becoming joys) but also redeem it. His paintings were a miraculous means by which Spencer would get himself to where all was holy, personal and at peace: to where he was at home in the universe. Like Christ's, his real triumph would lie not in a material kingdom but in a spiritual overcoming; like Christ (despite the agonies of the inevitable and perpetual confusions and frustrations of existence) he would find both meaning and liberation in his creativity, by finding himself in communion with God and Nature.

[T]o produce something which would make me walk with God.

I loved it all because it was all God and me, all the time.[14]

Spencer's vision amounted to a continuous procession in his mind: an unrolling pageant of material/spiritual sensations and expressions. It could overwhelm him but it also provided a magisterial transcendence, and he dedicated his life and art to its reproduction. His personal vision was ultimately individual and private.

The most exciting thing I ever came across is myself.[13]

I like my own life so much that I would like to cover every empty space on a wall with it.[15]

I don't want to lose sight of myself for a second.[2]

Artwork: compensation or fulfilment

Resurrection was a favoured subject of Spencer's and throughout his life he painted a number of works with this word in the title, set in places to which he felt he belonged, and which he loved; through the painting he was able to come to know the place even better, and also to express his love better. Thoughts of resurrection were never far from Spencer's mind, it seems, and the 'last day', when resurrection would take place, became an all encompassing theme, an umbrella concept for his artistic vision as a whole. What Spencer conceived of in a 'resurrection of the dead' was not necessarily physical so much as a becoming aware of the real meaning of life, and becoming alive to its enormous possibilities. Resurrections are displacements: awakenings to a state of realisation of the potentialities of heaven on earth which sex and love, joy and oneness (as against cruelty, 'othering', hate, fear, suspicion and lust for power) represent. Such an awakening or enlightenment could come to any person at any time, Spencer believed; moreover, after this 'last judgement', all would be 'acquitted' without punishment:

[A]ll things are redeemable in my opinion and I paint them in their redeemed state.[16]

Spencer's most ambitious goal was the representation in his art – and hence the emotional/spiritual accomplishment – of human salvation.

Firstly, in the Resurrections, is found a redeeming of Spencer's own life. His various 'loves and longings' are 'made whole', with the day-to-day viewpoint of his life being seen askance *sub specie aeternitatis*. Spencer draws together the various strands of his life, religious and secular, his associations with people and places, and his memories of their 'beloved ways and habits'. In particular, there is a reunion between Spencer and the important women in his life: his wives Hilda and Patricia, and close friends Daphne and Charlotte. A personal reconciliation with his first love (and continued closest friend), Hilda, figures repeatedly. Even though they were physically separated (by divorce and illness) for 20 years before her death, and for nine more years before his, Spencer continued 'conversing' with her in words and paint, and maintained a myth of their communication. An ultimate reconciliation between them was an act of faith for him. In his Resurrections, Spencer envisaged a general harmonising of relations between people, as well as a harmonising of his own life. Families and lovers, the quick and the dead, are reunited to engage in the heaven on earth of simple social and domestic activities, leisure and lovemaking. The resurrection is an occasion of surprise and wonderment. People are inspired by the new meaning in their life; there is a 'beautiful wholeness' as the fulfilment of all life's hopes and wishes comes about. People feel and share joy at meeting again, and at the peace that this brings. It is a time of love's triumph over discord and adversity, and of sublime truth; here is a realisation that, in love, people are in heaven.

What, then, may be said of the overall relationship between Spencer's artistry – his consciousness of his creative vision – and the way he lived his life, the control he was able to exert over it? Certainly, he was happiest when a coming together of life and vision was managed without personal suffering; but this was not always or easily the case. He suffered in the war, and through the regimentation of the army; he suffered the loss of Hilda and rejection by Patricia, and two stressful divorce proceedings; he suffered from the censorial atmosphere of a parochial England which left him frustrated from having to hide a frank depiction of self-exposure and sexual fantasy; he suffered from the dispersal of his art, a dependence on patronage, and an inability to secure any for his grander projects, and he was also short of money. And yet it seems that such was the strength of Spencer's personal vision that he was able to reconcile life and artistry despite these sufferings and thus to sustain his life project. Hell, Spencer once suggested, must be existing in a state of unimaginativeness and imperviousness to the spiritual. Surrounded by the imaginary world of his art and writings, this was something he never suffered; he lived his art and was pleased to do so.

Perhaps this is easiest to see in his relationship with Hilda. Hilda was probably the person to whom he felt closest in the world; in her he saw the same mental attitude to things as himself. Hilda became his great 'hand holder' and affirmer, the one who secured him and grounded him so that his imagination and emotion were stimulated. Indeed, his whole philosophy of love grew out of his love for Hilda and at one point Spencer felt that his written autobiography called for contributions from Hilda too: a hodge podge showing 'both our journeys'.

However, Spencer's self-intense nature made him turn their everyday relationship into something spiritual. His love for Hilda was as much sublime as earthly, and became more so:

> Hilda was the love I felt for what I looked at. She was the smoke coming from the factory chimneys. I want and need her in all my experience.[13]

His love united him not only to her, but to all creation and to God too; it bound all together for Spencer, affirming his existence and art. It grew so that it was impossible for him to separate Hilda from his vision, her presence in it seeming ancient and primordial. Increasingly, however, in spite of this, Spencer found himself and Hilda to be incompatible partners. Their preferred lifestyles drew them apart and their actual worlds were private ones; each could only approach the other from their respective lives. Indeed, it is arguable that Spencer found he could live with Hilda happily (and love her memory) only after divorcing her:

> Hilda: You are too much of an artist to have satisfactory relations with any women. That is the price you have to pay for your genius.

> Spencer: In spite of all I feel for you and my need for you, somewhere in me is an absence of love. I never have fulfilled love for another.[2]

Hilda becomes his phantasm and her image is more lovable than her person. Spencer concludes:

> [It is] incredible that you exist in the flesh![2]

There was also the Patricia question. Spencer at one stage wanted them both; Hilda: spiritual, domestic, thoughtful, considerate, sincere, complex, gauche, circumspect, intense; and Patricia: sophisticated, sexy, socially connected, elegant, stylish, vivid, lively, direct, forceful, superficial, teasing and opportunistic. The laws of England may not allow him two wives, but he would have two all the same; he would behave as he felt proper, irrespective of how others did. Certainly, he remonstrated, marriage was a private matter, whatever the law said. For Hilda and Patricia each gave him something necessary but different for the development of his artistic vision. He could be passionate, sincere and wholehearted to both: but Hilda retreated, and then Patricia did too. Which left Spencer and Hilda continually writing and reading letters to one another to mediate their loss; (exchanging letters had been their favoured form of communication and lovemaking from the start). As Hilda withdrew from his everyday life, Spencer found himself progressively able to idealise the figure Hilda represented for him. Her awkward personality could be made increasingly to conform to his artistic needs and to a position in his paintings' imagery; she joined the pantheon of personalities, real and imagined, contemporary and biblical, with which he was to populate the private world of his paintings. She is to be found there playing the role of youthful confidante, or comforting mother figure looming over a wondering Spencer like a form of protective covering. Having 'lost' the real Hilda through divorce and then death, Spencer developed their spiritual union to the point where she acts as his supportive ideal companion, Madonna and alter ego. Their erstwhile dialogue (always, perhaps, a matter more of contemporaneous monologues than of conversational give and take[2]) is now a self-dialogue which Spencer maintains within himself.

It might be argued that in constructing lovers (and others) largely in terms of his own imagination, Spencer's artistry served him primarily as a means of finding refuge from his personal difficulties; that the imaginary world of his art grew as his life's frustrations did, a means of vicarious living, justifying his actions and fulfilling his dreams. Support for this view could be drawn from Spencer's own words:

> [M]y desire to paint is caused by my being unable – or being incapable – of fulfilling my desires in life itself.[16]

Furthermore, some of Spencer's most poignant representations of domestic perfection – recreating his own marital harmony of the 1920s – were painted while attempting to divorce Hilda in the later 1930s. Does this not show that his artistic vision rose as his real life relationships plummeted? Yet, this is not the conclusion I would draw: Spencer's artistry was not as strategic or mannered as this, his art did not compensate for his life, it was the fulfilment of his life project. One's individual self, one's real spiritual self, Spencer was fond of claiming, is present everywhere. One way he explained this was by saying that it was because one was part of God, and wherever God was you were too. Another way was by saying that he, Spencer, was desirous to absorb everything in the

world into himself, to find himself to be a 'treasure island', and that this was
something of which all individuals were always capable. His creative impulse,
Spencer continued, was all-embracing: he possessed a voracious enjoyment in
looking at the world, dreaming it and recreating it. However much he dallied
with the trope of being in need of mothering, he was *au fond* self-reliant, and
gained a fierce, wild, self-sufficient happiness from painting alone. In the
'impregnable castle of his imagination',[2] Spencer had all that was necessary to
him; nothing he really needed could be either taken from him or given to him.
He wished for people to be there when he wanted to unburden himself but then
for him to be left alone in order to 'live my inner self'. Moreover, his vision, his
self, his appetite, he believed was unique to him and self-created:

> I know of nothing that I have ever done that I could say I did as a
> result of the love of God or because authorised by Him.[2]

This was why he was so chary of any suggestion of influences on his work: his
creation was pure, his work individual. His ambition too was great. He was aware
that the 'almost frightening candour' with which he revealed his originally perceived world 'without reserve'[18] was creating a personal iconography which challenged every contemporary English aesthetic norm, and he once admitted he was
in danger of becoming 'smug on success'.

Conclusion

Stanley Spencer wanted nothing less than to represent and realise a spiritual
redemption of the entire everyday world. Looking round him, in Cookham and
beyond, Spencer saw people, material objects, and practices possessed of 'the
sacred', of something transcendent. More than anything else this quickened his
sensibilities, and he desired to portray it – pictorially and verbally. Spencer felt that
through this portrayal he could make this presence something really known;
through his art he could present a paradisiacal reality where people shared a happy
and homely brotherhood with one another and their environment, and were
aware of their grace. Moreover, for Spencer, to compose this portrayal was to
become part of it: to live too in sacred, mysterious identification with the world 'in
the land of me'. His art was actually, personally, life-creating. In painting he
achieved union through the space of his canvas. And in this union, everything phe-
nomenal might be overcome, rescued and redeemed: everything past and present,
everything agreeable, disagreeable and mortifying, misfortuned, friendly and tragic.

It was not by chance that Stanley often pictured himself and his characters
walking with Christ, and described himself as part of God. Stanley was a Christ-
like prophet to himself:

> [P]ainting with me was the crowning of an already elected king.[13]

> [I am] a new kind of Adam, and joy is the means by which I name
> things.[2]

In transposing his friends and lovers and himself, Cookham, Port Glasgow, Leonard
Stanley, Hampstead, and so on, into the imagined worlds of his figurative art, he
was able to displace, represent and replace the whole world in a quasi-divine way.

His message of love – ambitious, arrogant, certain, strange – might sit uneasily alongside English politeness and reserve but one day it would be acclaimed the truth. Meantime, his metaphysic was a source of wellbeing and something with which his 'non-artistic projects', such as these were, had to come to terms:

> Stanley: [I]t has been my way to make things as far as I am able to – fit me.[19]

> Hilda: You would reckon to shape your own destiny, and therefore forcing things and riding right over them is part of your outlook. To you that seems right, to take the matter in your own hands and shape it as you will.[13]

It would be my conclusion that weighing up the evidence of his life this was something which Stanley Spencer succeeded in effecting. The power of his imagination and the discipline with which he lived it made Stanley his own man. His artistic vision amounted to a life project whereby he acquired the genius to inhabit successfully a world of his own construal. He related to a social environment created in his own image.

Acknowledgements

The final drafting of this paper took place while I was a Visiting Professor at the School of Anthropology, Geography, and Environmental Studies, University of Melbourne. I am very grateful to members of that institution, in particular Professor Andrew Dawson. I am also grateful to the guest editors of the special issue of *Medical Humanities* and the anonymous reviewers for their constructive commentaries.

References

1 Rapport NJ (1997) *Transcendent Individual: towards a liberal and literary anthropology*. Routledge, London.
2 Collis M (1962) *Stanley Spencer*. Harvill, London.
3 Emerson RW (1981) *The Portable Emerson*. Penguin, Harmondsworth.
4 Kateb G (1991) Introduction: exile, alienation and estrangement. *Soc Res*. **58**: 135–8.
5 Rapport NJ, Dawson A (1998) *Home and Movement: a polemic. Migrants of identity: perceptions of home in a world of movement*. Berg, Oxford.
6 Cohen AP (1994) *Self Consciousness*. Routledge, London.
7 Schuetz A (1972) *The Phenomenology of the Social World*. Heinemann, London.
8 Jackson M (1996) *Introduction: phenomenology, radical empiricism, and 'anthropological critique'. Things as they are*. Indiana University Press, Bloomington, IN.
9 Eves R (1998) *The Magical Body*. Harwood Academic, Amsterdam.
10 Sartre J-P (1972) *The Psychology of Imagination*. Citadel, New York.
11 Rapport NJ (2003) *I Am Dynamite: an alternative anthropology of power*. Routledge, London.
12 Nietzsche F (1994) *Human. All too human*. Penguin, Harmondsworth.
13 Pople K (1991) *Stanley Spencer*. Collins, London.
14 Bell K (1992) *Stanley Spencer*. Phaidon, London.
15 Glew A (ed) (2001) *Stanley Spencer: letters and writing*. Tate, London.
16 Robinson D (1994) *Stanley Spencer*. Phaidon, London.
17 Spencer S (1991) *The Apotheosis of Love*. Barbican Art Gallery, London.
18 Rothenstein E (1945) *Stanley Spencer*. Phaidon, London.
19 Arts Council of Great Britain. *Stanley Spencer*. Macle, Glasgow.

Chapter 2

Constructions of self: ethical overtones in surprising locations

Elizabeth A Kinsella

While conceptions of 'self' may seem self-explanatory and often appear to be taken as self-evident within health professions, the literature concerning how the self is constructed has been burgeoning in other fields. Various philosophers and theorists have, in recent years, drawn attention to conflicting conceptions of the self, and raised this as an important domain of concern at both a theoretical and practical level. Conceptions of the 'self' vary, from interpretations that focus on 1) the unitary rationalistic subject of the enlightenment project, to 2) decentred and fragmented poststructural and postmodern subjects, to 3) narrative and dialogic views. These three perspectives are considered in the first section, followed by discussions that highlight ethical issues revealed when one attends to a narrative and dialogic conception of the self.

I argue that health practitioners possess significant power to either affirm or demean the individual's conceptions of self, and harm can occur when practitioners fail to recognise this power. Further, subtle ethical issues with respect to how relationship and language may be employed to wield power in healthcare practice are considered. The question of how this power can be ethically used in healthcare practice is raised.

This chapter adopts a hermeneutic approach.[1-3] Ferraris[4] views hermeneutics as 'the art of interpretation as transformation' and contrasts it with a view of theory as 'contemplation of eternal essences unalterable by the observer'. A hermeneutic approach seeks understanding rather than explanation, acknowledges the situated location of interpretation, recognises that language and history are both conditions and limitations of understanding, views inquiry as conversation, and is comfortable with ambiguity.[1-3] For Gadamer[5] hermeneutics 'is entrusted with all that is unfamiliar and strikes us as significant'. From this perspective the meaning of a text is not to be compared with an immovably and obstinately fixed point of view, rather 'to understand a text means always to apply it to ourselves and to know that, even if it must always be understood in different ways it is still the same text presenting itself to us in these different ways'.[2] A hermeneutic approach is open to the ambiguous nature of textual analysis and invites a polyphony of perspectives into the conversation – therefore perspectives that may not otherwise come into dialogue with one another and that cross traditional borders are brought together in conversation. A hermeneutic attitude is revealed in this study through a posture of conversation, as invitation to reflect on the tensions that arise in the discussion.

Constructions of 'self': three perspectives

Unitary self

The unitary self of the enlightenment project has been depicted as presupposing an essence at the heart of the individual which is unique, fixed and coherent and which makes her or him what she or he is.[6] This individuated rational self – frequently attributed to Descartes and his famous dictum 'I think, therefore I am' – perceives itself through self-reflection. Cognition, from this perspective, appears as a type of inner contemplation, conducted by the solitary meditator.[7] Such a conception presupposes a self who experiences the world independently of the language and discourse in which statements about the world are made.[8] Also, the focus on the individual is distinct from older dialogic views of existence.[7] This unitary, rational self, a knowing subject who comes to know itself through self-reflection, is the conception that implicitly informs much humanist discourse.

Fragmented and decentred self

In contrast, postmodern and poststructuralist views posit a conception of a fragmented, decentred self. Postmodern writers question whether the self is unified, singular and self-determining, highlighting, as Lyotard[9] does, that each self exists in a fabric of relations. Poststructuralism proposes a self that is precarious, contradictory and in process, constantly being reconstituted in discourse each time we think or speak.[6] Foucault, for example,[10] argues that as subjects there is no single position from which we can be empowered but only particular discursive positions within power/knowledge formations. For Foucault, subjects are constituted in discourse.

In Lacan's view individuals are constituted as divided subjects,[11,12] split between the subject of being (the self identified as 'me') and the subject of language (the self identified as 'I').[12] The 'subject of being' located in the imaginary order cannot be conflated with the 'subject of speech' located in the symbolic order. As Lacan points out: 'I identify myself in language, but only by losing myself in it like an object.'[12] Lacan draws attention to the separation between the subject in 'being' and the subject in 'speech' and seeks to differentiate rather than conflate the two.[12] Without this distinction, it is assumed that we are able to stand over against ourselves, and our practices, as if we are knowing subjects standing in relation to an object; yet postmodern and poststructural theories call this assumption into question.[12]

From a postmodern/poststructuralist point of view, curricula in healthcare education that fail to problematise the modern notion of an individuated, self-transparent consciousness, fully in control of itself, are problematic. Postmodern and poststructuralist thinkers contend that the self is more than cognitive and rational minds ruling bodies; the self is also constituted and reconstituted in relationship and language. This is a conversation that I suggest requires considerably more attention than it has received to date in healthcare professions. Postmodern and poststructural perspectives invite those working in health education to become reflexive about the conceptions of self that subtly pervade professional preparatory programmes.

Narrative and dialogic self

An alternative view of the self, which is responsive to issues of relationship and language yet maintains the agency of the individual, is a *narrative and dialogic* one. Such a conception offers promise for healthcare education and illuminates ethical imperatives that may otherwise remain invisible.

Numerous theorists have suggested that narrative is a fundamental way of attributing meaning in our lives,[13,14] and that constructing stories about the self is linked to the construction of self-identity.[13,15,16] Lindemann Nelson[15] captures this idea eloquently:

> Personal identities consist of a connective tissue of narratives – some constant, others shifting over time – which we weave around the features of our selves and our lives that matter most to us.

The significant things I've done and experienced, my more important characteristics, the roles and relationships I care about most, the values that matter most to me – these form the relatively stable points around which I construct the narratives that constitute the sense I make of myself. The stories of my connection to these things over time are explanatory: they explain to me who I am and it's this that is my own contribution to my personal identity.

Similarly, Polkinghorne[16] highlights the narrative achievement of personal identity as follows: we achieve our personal identities and self-concept through the use of the narrative configuration, and make our existence into a whole by understanding it as an expression of a single unfolding and developing story. We are in the middle of our stories and cannot be sure how they will end; we are constantly having to revise the plot as new events are added to our lives. Self, then, is not a static thing or a substance, but a configuring of personal events into an historical unity which includes not only what one has been but also anticipations of what one will be.

As well as acknowledging the individual's role in constructing his or her self-concept through narrative configuration and revision, European philosopher Richard Kearney[17] calls for attention to a dialogic dimension. Such an account recognises that a narrative configuration of the self involves not only a reflexive relationship of self to self, but also a relationship of self to other.[18] This relationship of self to other may be referred to as intersubjectivity – a *relation* and *response* between the subjectivity of the self and the subjectivity of the other. This interanimation or intersubjectivity is achieved through dialogue, and draws on the vehicle of language.

The word dialogue comes from the Greek word *dialogos*.[19]

> Logos means 'the word', or…the 'meaning of the word'. And dia means 'through'… The picture or image that this derivation suggests is of a stream of meaning flowing among and through us and between us.[19]

In physicist/philosopher, David Bohm's view,[19] dialogue is a process of direct face-to-face encounter that insists on facing the inconvenient messiness of daily, corporeal lived experience. This dialogic dimension is an invitation to test the viability of traditional definitions of what it means to be human and collectively to explore the prospect of an enhanced humanity.[20]

Similarly, philosopher Charles Taylor[21] argues that the general feature of human life is its fundamentally dialogical character, and that identities are formed in open dialogue. For Taylor the formation of identity crucially depends on one's dialogical relations with others. He writes: 'My discovering my identity doesn't mean that I work it out in isolation but that I negotiate it through dialogue, partly overtly, partly internalised, with others.'[21] Taylor suggests that we become full human agents, capable of understanding ourselves, and hence of defining an identity, through our acquisition of rich human languages of expression. These include not only words but languages of art, gesture, love, and the like. Yet we do not acquire the languages needed for self-definition on our own, rather we are introduced to them through exchanges with others who matter to us. The genesis of the human mind is in this sense not 'monological', not something each accomplishes on his or her own, but dialogical.[21] Taylor notes that dialogue invokes both agreement and struggle, as 'our identities are formed in dialogue with others, in agreement or struggle with their recognition of us'.[21] Dialogical relationships carry weight in our constructions of self as 'we are all aware how identity can be formed or malformed in our contact with significant others'.[21]

The dialogic nature of human life is highlighted as an important complement to traditional conceptions of narrative. The achievement of identity is viewed as both an individual and an intersubjective event. Such a recognition raises ethical issues for practitioners in healthcare, which are elaborated in subsequent sections of this chapter.

The work of European philosopher Richard Kearney and Russian philosopher Mikhail Bakhtin also support a narrative *and* dialogic conception of the self. Philosopher Richard Kearney[17] notes that a narrative *and* dialogic perspective retains the agency of the practitioner while taking intersubjectivity and language into account. He argues that following postmodernism and poststructuralism, theorists must reinvent a genuine narrative subject. He proposes a narrative self prepared to work through the pain of the past in dialogue with its 'others'. Kearney calls for 'a postdeconstructionist subject, able to carry out acts of semantic innovation (poetics) and just judgment (ethics)'.[17] He believes it is possible to take on the postmodern assaults on the unitary subject without dispensing with all notions of selfhood. Kearney argues that 'without some sense of self there can be no sense of the other-than-self', yet paradoxically 'the shortest route from self to self is always through the other'.[17] In contrast to the Cartesian perspective, he argues that meaning 'does not originate within the narrow chambers of its own subjectivity, but emerges as a response to the other, as radical intersubjectivity'.[22]

Bakhtin's thinking also supports a reinvigoration of a narrative and dialogic conception of the self.[23] Bakhtin contends that we exist through 'the borrowed axiological light of otherness',[24] highlighting the intersubjective and dialogic nature of existence. Bakhtin proposes acting agents whose ethical actions are constituted in particular, unique acts. Bakhtin believes that our lives can be consciously comprehended only in *answerability*. By answerability he refers to our ability to take responsibility for our acts (including thoughts). In *Toward a Philosophy of the Act*, Bakhtin writes:

> My entire life as a whole can be considered as a single complex act or deed that I perform.[25]

An answerable life, according to Bakhtin, is one in which there is 'no alibi' for Being. He says that:

> A life that has fallen away from answerability cannot have a philosophy:
> it is by its very principle, fortuitous and incapable of being rooted.[25]

Answerability invokes 'the necessity of dialogue between two people who come into an event with specific horizons of meaning, and who then act to answer others' actions'.[26] Bakhtin's 'answerable' subject, then, reflects a narrative and dialogic self. In this view the individual is answerable to another, meaning is creatively reconstituted and shifted through dialogue, yet the individual maintains a sense of agency. The self in this conception is not reduced to a pawn constructed solely by external forces, yet neither is the individual a solitary, self-contained being. Thus, Bakhtin's views depict an evolution from the 'unitary self' and the 'fragmented self' to support a conception of a narrative *and* dialogic self.

In summary, a narrative *and* dialogic notion of self engages with the spaces between the conceptions of a modern unitary essential and individuated self (known through self-reflection) *and* a postmodern decentred and fragmented self (constituted in discourse and social relations). Such a perspective recognises the achievement of personal identities and self-concept through the use of the narrative configuration, viewing the self not as a static thing or a substance, but rather as an active agent who configures personal events into a historical unity; while also recognising the dialogic nature of identity and therefore the central role of intersubjectivity (response to/from the other) and language (the vehicle for such response) in its configuration.

In light of a narrative and dialogic conception of self, ethical considerations arise which I consider in the following two sections. In the first section, I suggest that harm can occur in practice when healthcare practitioners fail to recognise the power they wield with respect to relational and intersubjective considerations that influence identity. I argue that health practitioners possess significant power to either affirm or demean the identity of the other. In the second section, I seek to reveal ethical issues with respect to how language and discourse may be employed in healthcare practice, and to highlight ethical imperatives for a thoughtful consideration of how this power is used in practice.

Ethical relationship and intersubjectivity

What occurs in practice when we fail to consider the intersubjective or dialogic nature of experience in our theoretical constructs? With respect to client relationships, Taylor and White[27] note that while practitioner reflection opens up the possibility of a more uncertain, ambiguous and complex world, it has the potential to close much of this down again. By freezing practitioners' accounts, as true representations of what happened, practitioner reflection can unintentionally obscure client perspectives. Such a privileging of the practitioner perspective can be dangerous.

In healthcare practice, the practitioner's experience and constructions become very powerful, and given that the professional is often already in a position of power with respect to his or her client, the professional's constructions may occlude the experience of the 'other' and may even disempower clients. This certainly does not call for an exclusion of attention to practitioner reflection, which is certainly a step in a progressive direction. Rather, I suggest that it calls for greater attention to the intersubjective and dialogic nature of experience in practice. This includes attention to and discussion about the ways in which clients construct meanings, and the creation of environments that foster dialogic communication. I suggest that a humble recognition is required that individuals are 'co-creators' of meaning within practice environments – even and most particularly when one party is privileged with the social status of 'expert'. Once again philosophers Charles Taylor, Richard Kearney, Mikhail Bakhtin and others offer perspectives that contribute to this conversation.

Taylor[21] suggests that an original identity needs (and is vulnerable to) the recognition given or withheld by significant others. According to Taylor, equal recognition is not just the appropriate mode for a healthy democratic society: its refusal can inflict damage on those who are denied it. The projecting of an inferior or demeaning image on another can actually distort and oppress, to the extent that it is interiorised. People's beliefs bear directly on the construction and misconstruction of personal identities, and it is that aspect of oppression that is of concern.[15] Practitioners have considerable power to grant or withhold recognition of significant others and to grant or withhold spaces in which divergent accounts of meaning and identity can be expressed and tested. Acknowledgement of this power and consideration of its ethical use within professional relationships is crucially important.

Kearney[22] draws on continental philosopher Emmanuel Levinas[28] to demonstrate that, in ethical relationships, the face of the other calls out to us for response before epistemological and ontological concerns. Levinas calls this the ethical relation of the 'face to face'. Another in need makes the ethical demand on me: where are you? We are responsible for the suffering of the other in that face-to-face moment.[22] With respect to healthcare practice, to simply reflect on one's own interpretations without a consideration of the 'face of the other' and an acknowledgement of the 'other's' construction of meaning, in light of one's own, raises ethical questions. As mentioned earlier Kearney believes that meaning emerges as a response to the other, as *radical intersubjectivity*.

Bakhtin's thoughts on ethical relationship also provide a useful way to think about intersubjectivity. Bakhtin suggests that in ethical relationship we as individuals are answerable to another through our non-alibi in Being.[25] He writes:

> To live from within oneself does not mean to live for oneself, but means to be an answerable participant from within oneself, to affirm one's compellent, actual non-alibi in Being.[25]

Bakhtin points out that without an adequate consideration of human encounters, we are in danger of confronting 'the other as a thing, as a raw material to be objectified and manipulated in accordance with an egocentric self interest'.[29] This is opposed to his view of the other 'as a unique and singular being, in which a dialogical relation is reciprocal and mutually enriching'.[29] According to Bakhtin[30] monologic approaches that centre only on the individual's construction of meaning deny the dialogic nature of existence, refuse to recognise the responsibility of the addressee, and pretend to be the 'last word'. Bakhtin believes that meaning is always a becoming, the result of the dialogic give and take between the inside and the outside, the self and the world, the self and the other. In his view meaning is intertextual and dialogic.

The preceding discussion raises many issues. As opposed to separate individuated human beings, as in the unitary conception of self, the self is portrayed as vulnerable to, but also informed and potentially liberated by, others. In this way, the role of intersubjectivity in the constitution of identity is highlighted. One potential implication of 'constructions of self' that exclude a focus on intersubjectivity is the danger of creating environments that unintentionally demean or oppress, that treat clients or co-workers as objects of our reflections – that is, as things.

If meaning is indeed intersubjective and dialogically constituted, the practitioner is called to be answerable to the 'other'. This can be a challenge, particularly in healthcare environments that promote practitioners as experts, and that emphasise 'evidence' and 'efficiency'. To be answerable to another demands that one must not be fearful of showing one's weakness; it demands humility and openness as opposed to pride and arrogance. Such a view runs contrary to many hierarchical and expert-centred environments. For instance, if one shows humility and openness it can be perceived as self-doubt, as lack of confidence, as 'not knowing'. I suggest that this is an important area of consideration in professional environments, and particularly in health profession environments. How can we promote cultures that invite openness, dialogue and responsiveness as opposed to monologic or arrogant approaches to healthcare?

A central question raised for me is whether health professional education goes far enough in the promotion of ethical dialogical relationships that acknowledge intersubjective dimensions in professional practice, and whether the call to 'professionalism' carries with it the danger of treating service users and colleagues as simply objects of practitioner reflections and constructions.

I suggest that more attention to intersubjective elements, with respect to conceptions of how the self is constructed, is warranted in health professional education.

Ethical issues in language and discourse

Ethical issues relative to language and discourse are revealed when a narrative and dialogic view of the self is considered. Rich[31] highlights the power of language, noting that it is the vehicle through which people name, describe and depict, and that through its corruption, language can also be used to manage our perceptions. Indeed, language has the power to organise our thought and experience and to frame the issues to which we address our attention.[32] Language then has a constitutive moral relation to its objects.[33] When such an understanding of language is applied to practice, the question of *who* frames the issues and whose version of reality holds sway is raised. Indeed, the potential to silence certain versions of reality through language is reflected in Cixous's and Calle-Gruber's insight that 'all narratives tell one story in place of another story'.[34]

In contrast to a non-problematic realist view of language, Foucault[35] is concerned with discourse as a system of representation. His main concern is with a broad macro-level analysis of discursive systems, and the relations of such systems to issues of power, as opposed to micro-level language analysis.[36] In Foucault's[35] view, discourse 'creates a field of knowledge by defining what is possible to say and think, declaring the bases for deciding what is true and authorising certain people to speak while making others silent or less authoritative'.[35] Gee[37,38] points out that discourses can be seen as ideological because they involve a set of values and viewpoints in terms of which one must speak and act, at least while one is in the discourse; otherwise one does not count as being in it.

Professional discourses (fields of knowledge) operate within particular professions, within disciplines, and within various institutions. Although often unacknowledged, professional discourses influence the manner in which practitioners act. Discursive regimes are linked to power, in that 'expert' practitioners can claim cognitive authority over the stories of practice. 'Cognitive authority' is a term coined by feminist philosopher Kathryn Pyne Addelson.[39] It refers to the authority to have one's descriptions of the world taken seriously, believed or accepted generally as truth. In professional practice, the discourses of professionals are frequently granted cognitive authority over the reports of others, and those of more powerful disciplines are often granted greater cognitive authority than those of less powerful groups. Rich[40] highlights the capacity of those with cognitive authority to silence other stories and points out the consequent potential for what she calls psychic disequilibrium. She writes:

> When someone with the authority of a teacher, say, describes the world and you are not in it, there is a moment of psychic disequilibrium, as if you looked into a mirror and saw nothing.[40]

Frye[41] describes a dominant position: one that excludes the other, takes one's own standpoint as central, one's own needs, opinions, desires and projects as the salient ones, and one's experience and understanding as what is the case.[15] Frye points out that oppressive master discourses commonly construct the identities of others from the perspective of the arrogant eye, dismissing or degrading what does not bear directly on their value to the dominant group. A failure to become conscious of the tendency to assimilate such 'authoritative discourses' into one's or one's client's identity is a danger in professional practice.

Whereas control over discourse is a vital source of power, it is important to note that there are limits to this control because meanings are fluid and can be reworked to resist domination.[42,43] Thus, both practitioners and clients have the capacity to actively resist or struggle with the meanings ensconced in authoritative discourses. Frye[41] has recognised that not all practitioners adopt the arrogant gaze highlighted above. Frye counters the 'arrogant eye' with a 'loving eye', one that confers the cognitive authority withheld by the arrogant gaze, such that discursive accounts that fall outside of the master discourse are not delegitimated.[15]

As an example, feminist philosopher Susan Wendell[44] relays the story of Gloria Murphy, a woman who experienced acute dizziness, numbness in the legs, inability to walk at times, double vision, bladder, kidney and bowel trouble. During most of the five years between the onset of her symptoms and her diagnosis of multiple sclerosis she was told by the Mayo clinic, and others, that she had 'housewife's syndrome' and needed to get busy and away from the children to feel better. The cognitive authority of this master discourse caused her to engage in extensive volunteer work and activities, despite frequent rehospitalisations, and to doubt her own strong feeling that something was very wrong. When she was diagnosed she was elated, the response being the result of being rid of a terrible conflict, between what Gloria felt and what the master discourse demanded that she believe about herself. Perhaps a 'loving gaze' could have helped Gloria to acknowledge and affirm the authority of her experience.

Once again ethically important issues arise. In the health professions, explicitly acknowledging the nature of discursive systems and reflecting upon the implications of powerful discourses with respect to the construction of identity becomes important. Another important issue is the imperative to critique dominant discourses and to recognise their power to legitimate who is permitted to name the values or problems of practice and who is granted cognitive authority.

This question of whose version of the world is told and whose is silenced is an important one. The potential of discursive systems to contribute to the constructions of identity, to suppress certain accounts, and to infuse others with authority reveals an important ethical dimension of practice that is not often considered in health professional education yet which influences the manner in which practitioners behave.

Conclusion: constructions of self and ethical practice

How one wields relational and discursive power is an ethical matter. Therefore, conceptions of the self that consider intersubjectivity and language have profound implications for ethical practice. Chapman[43] advocates not a universalising and objectifying moral code but a constantly evolving ethical practice grounded in the everyday, in which the practitioner is conscious of and attempts to wield power in an ethical manner. Such an ethical practice is informed by the 'loving eye' posited by Frye,[41] a gaze that recognises the cognitive authority of discourses beyond its own. I suggest that attention to the problematic nature of intersubjectivity, discourse and language in professional practice are important sites for ethical discussions in healthcare fields.

Conceptions of how the 'self' is 'constructed' – while seemingly abstract and theoretical – are, I contend, immensely practical. Such conceptions inform the ethical considerations that carry weight in our day-to-day interactions and behaviours in practice. The manner in which health practitioners use or misuse relationships and language to construct 'others', to construct versions of reality, to construct meaning and to wield cognitive authority has immense implications for day-to-day life in healthcare environments. I suggest that a narrative and dialogic conceptualisation of the 'self' allows for a dialogue about these issues, and holds much promise for the education and practice of health professionals of the future. Yet I recognise that fostering such a view is not without challenges; given that modernist notions appear to underpin current practices, decisions about conceptions of self are not widely recognised as ethically significant, and tensions are created in environments that promote practitioners as experts.

Nonetheless, the elaboration of a narrative and dialogic conception of the self, and the study of intersubjectivity and language use as they relate to power, offer promising locations for further study, as well as profound sites for the consideration of ethical imperatives for practice in the health professions.

Acknowledgement

This work was supported in part by The Social Sciences and Humanities Research Council of Canada.

References

1 Gadamer HG (1976) *Philosophical Hermeneutics* [trans Linge D]. University of California Press, Berkeley.

2 Gadamer HG (1996) *Truth and Method* [trans Weinsheimer J, Marshall D]. Continuum, New York.

3 Jardine D (1992) Reflections on education, hermeneutics, and ambiguity: hermeneutics as a restoring of life to its original difficulty. In: W Pinar and W Reynolds (eds).

Understanding Curriculum as Phenomenological and Deconstructed Text. Teachers College Press, New York.

4 Ferraris M (1996) *History of Hermeneutics* [trans Somigli L]. Humanities Press, Atlantic Highlands, NY.

5 Gadamer HG (1992) Interview: writing and the living voice. In: D Misgeld and G Nicholson (eds). *Hans-Georg Gadamer on Education, Poetry and History*. State University of New York Press, New York.

6 Weedon C (1987) *Feminist Practice and Poststructural Theory*. Blackwell, Cambridge.

7 Sandywell B (1999) Specular grammar: the visual rhetoric of modernity. In: I Heywood and B Sandywell (eds). *Interpreting Visual Culture: explorations in the hermeneutics of the visual*. Routledge, London.

8 Smith D (1999) *Writing the Social*. University of Toronto Press, Toronto.

9 Lyotard JF (1979) *The Postmodern Condition: a report on knowledge* [trans Bennington G, Massumi B]. Manchester University Press, Manchester.

10 Foucault M (1980) *Power/knowledge: selected interviews and other writings 1972–1977* [trans Bouchard D, Simon S]. Pantheon Books, New York.

11 Lacan J (1977) *Ecrits: a selection* [trans Sheridan A]. Tavistock, London.

12 Carson T (1997) Reflection and its resistances: teacher education as a living practice. In: T Carson and D Sumara (eds). *Action Research as a Living Practice*. Peter Lang, New York.

13 Bruner J (1990) *Acts of Meaning*. Harvard University Press, Cambridge, MA.

14 Garro L and Mattingly C (2000) Narrative as construct and construction. *Narrative and the Cultural Construction of Illness and Healing*. University of California Press, Berkeley.

15 Nelson HL (2001) *Damaged Identities: narrative repair*. Cornell University Press, Ithaca, NY.

16 Polkinghorne DE (1988) *Narrative Knowing and the Human Sciences*. State University of New York Press, New York.

17 Kearney R (2003) *Strangers, Gods, and Monsters: interpreting otherness*. Routledge, London.

18 Ricoeur P (1992) *Oneself as Another*. University of Chicago Press, Chicago.

19 Bohm D (1996) *On Dialogue*. Routledge, London.

20 Nichol L (1996) Foreword. In: D Bohn. *On Dialogue*. Routledge, London.

21 Taylor C (1992) *The Ethics of Authenticity*. Harvard University Press, Cambridge, MA.

22 Kearney R (1988) *The Wake of Imagination*. Routledge, London.

23 Bakhtin M (1981) *The Dialogic Imagination* [trans Emerson C, Holquist M]. University of Texas Press, Austin, TX.

24 Bakhtin M (1990) *Art and Answerability* [trans Liapunov V, Brostrom K]. University of Texas Press, Austin, TX.

25 Bakhtin M (1993) *Toward a Philosophy of the Act*. University of Texas Press, Austin, TX.

26 Bender C (1998) Bakhtinian perspective on 'everyday life' sociology. In: M Bell and M Gardiner (eds). *Bakhtin and the Human Sciences*. Sage, London.

27 Taylor C and White S (2000) *Practising Reflexivity in Health and Welfare: making knowledge*. Open University Press, Buckingham.

28 Levinas E (1969) *Totality and Infinity*. Dusquesne University Press, Pittsburgh.

29 Gardiner M (1999) Bakhtin and the metaphorics of perception. In: I Heywood and B Sandywell (eds). *Interpreting Visual Culture: explorations in the hermeneutics of the visual*. Routledge, London.

30 Bakhtin M (1994) *The Bakhtin Reader*. Edward Arnold, London.

31 Rich A (2001) *Arts of the Possible*. WW Norton and Co, New York.

32 Lather P (1991) *Getting Smart: feminist research and pedagogy with/in the postmodern*. Routledge, New York.

33 Sandywell B (1996) *Reflexivity and the Crisis of Western Reason: logological investigations*. Routledge, London.

34 Cixous H and Calle-Gruber M (1997) *Rootprints: memory and life writing* [trans Prenowitz E]. Routledge, New York.

35 Foucault M (1974) *The Archaeology of Knowledge*. Tavistock, London.

36 Hall S (2001) Foucault: power, knowledge and discourse. In: M Wetherell, S Taylor and S Yates (eds). *Discourse Theory and Practice*. Sage, London.

37 Gee JP (1991) What is literacy? In: C Mitchell and K Weiler (eds). *Rewriting Literacy: culture and the discourse of the other*. Bergin & Garvey, New York.

38 Gee JP (1999) *An Introduction to Discourse Analysis: theory and method*. Routledge, London.

39 Addelson KP (1983) The man of professional wisdom. In: S Harding and M Hintikka (eds). *Discovering Reality*. D Reidel, Boston.

40 Rich A (1989) Invisibility in academe. In: R Rosaldo (ed). *Culture and Truth: the remaking of social analysis*. Beacon Press, Boston.

41 Frye M (1983) *The Politics of Reality*. Crossing, Freedom, CA.

42 Chapman V (2003) On 'knowing one's self' self writing, power and ethical practice: reflections from an adult educator. *Studies in the Education of Adults*. **35**: 35–53.

43 Wetherall M (2001) Themes in discourse research. In: M Wetherell, S Taylor and S Yates (eds). *Discourse Theory and Practice*. Sage, London.

44 Wendell S (1996) *The Rejected Body: feminist philosophical reflections on disability*. Routledge, New York.

Chapter 3

Some body wants to be normal: an account of an HIV narrative

Anabelle Mooney

> For us, the human body defines, by natural right, the space of origin and of distribution of disease: a space whose lines, volumes, surfaces, and routes are laid down, in accordance with a now familiar geometry, by the anatomical atlas.[1]

> What happens to my body happens to my life.[2]

So much recent scholarship has focused, rightly, on the social construction of illness that we may be in danger of forgetting that illness is in the body. Bodies carry things that are illnesses. Some of these things are themselves bodies in another sense – viruses, bacteria. Sometimes our bodies are at dis-ease. Something is not working the way it is supposed to be.[3] Further, constructions of illness are written on the body.

> Our bodies describe the story of our lives for better or for worse.[4]

Sometimes, the body has to be spoken for. Its story is not always legible, that is, clear and transparent. A common way of telling the story of the body is in the form of medical and biological language. Such a story might better be called a description or an explanation. In terms of allopathic medicine, it is clear that science is just another way of telling a story and then acting on the basis of this. The notion that science is objective, true and singular has long been under attack.[5-9] Science is, however, still the primary framing device for illness, even though other perspectives are increasingly included. Historically speaking, the scientific framing of HIV was dependent on more individual narratives. In particular relation to the early days of HIV, Patton notes:

> In the first few years of the epidemic…[m]any men (and some women) willingly gave evidence of their illness and of their life, describing symptoms and answering long epidemiological questionnaires about the intimate details of rich and complex sex lives… But once the disease had been wrested out of the discourse of people living with AIDS, once HIV was discovered and could be made to perform in the laboratory without homosexual bodies, science no longer wanted to hear that discourse.[10]

Before scientific theory comes the story. When the scientific theory is able to explain and predict, individual narratives are no longer required as a starting point. They become merely exemplars of the theory that they informed.

John's story

This chapter examines a body carrying the human immunodeficiency virus (HIV) and the resulting narratives. It is a particular case: one person who regards his body as the carrier for more than just an illness. For reasons of confidentiality, I will call this person John. John does not consider himself normal, and adjusts his body to the very normality from which he is alienated. It is not the qualified gaze which John fears,[1] but rather, the way in which people may alter their gaze once they know what they cannot even see. What is feared is the way in which others will write his illness on his body. While this is certainly a social construction, it finds expression physically in an active dissembling of a bodily state. Treichler finds 'Turner's postulates' useful in 'rewriting the AIDS text':[11]

> (1) disease is a language; (2) the body is a representation; and (3) medicine is a political practice.[12]

The gaze John fears is the one he has constructed and apprehends. Lacan writes of 'the pre-existence of a gaze – I see only from one point, but in my existence I am looked at from all sides... We are beings who are looked at, in the spectacle of the world'.[13] In short, John sees himself being seen. This is neither an epiphany nor an actual event. Simply, he already sees himself as he fears others would see him. As his body carries HIV he cannot see his body as normal. As a consequence, he cannot see himself as normal.

The narrative examined in this chapter is also an explanation, one in which the body is central. The HIV body cannot speak for itself unless one has access to bodily fluids and scientific measures. The story that the narrator, John, tells, the subject of this chapter, is very different from a medical account of HIV and AIDS.

HIV is in fact written on the body at the level of DNA through RNA transcription.[*]

Joughin notes that HIV is 'a retrovirus which works its wiles in reverse transcriptions, breaks codes, and en(s)crypts itself within a body/text which can no longer distinguish *inside* from *outside*' (my emphasis).[15] The AIDS discourse is itself an epidemic. Joughin reminds us that:

> Just as AIDS is a writerly sickness writ large, an epidemic of, and in, signification, the skewed parameters and loaded positionalities of its reinscription function within a complex discursive field in which many reactional and entrenched narratives already intersect. In short, we need to remember that the signifier 'AIDS' is wielded as much in silent domination as in signification.[15]

HIV, however, is not, perhaps, the usual sort of illness.[16] In the case of HIV (until AIDS or opportunistic infections), there is no visible sickness as such. Herzlich affirms a relationship between illness and effect such that:

> The individual evaluates his condition not according to its intrinsic manifestations, but according to its effects.[17]

---

[*] For a provirus to produce new viruses, RNA copies must be made that can be read by the host cell's protein-making machinery. These copies are called messenger RNA (mRNA), and production of mRNA is called transcription, a process that involves the host cell's own enzymes. Viral genes in concert with the cellular machinery control this process: the tat gene, for example, encodes a protein that accelerates transcription. Genomic RNA is also transcribed for later incorporation in the budding virion.[14]

HIV is not a serious illness in the asymptomatic person in terms of 'intrinsic manifestations'. In terms of 'effects', however, the story is quite different. HIV is more appropriately a 'condition'. It is a condition which influences the way of telling and living the body, which includes relations with others.[17]

Background

The research background to this chapter is important in both a general and particular way. Over the past three years I have interviewed and spoken to dozens of positive people and professionals working in advocacy, care and support organisations. One thing is clear: every positive experience is different. Naturally there are some points of intersection in terms of difficulties with, for example, opportunistic infections and drug regimes, and family and relationships. Just when I thought I had heard it all, however, I would be surprised.

I am not suggesting that nothing at all can be said about HIV in general. Rather, in this instance I want to focus on an individual and (among my respondents) unique interpretation of the self as positive. The individual in this case draws largely on public narratives from the mass media of the mid-1980s. Now, they would be considered stereotypes. These representations of HIV have, however, been internalised by John, while at the same time being attributed to a generalised other. Whether this is because his diagnosis occurred in that period or because he accepts these narratives as true is beside the point (though I would opt for the latter). He can be understood as being trapped in a now dated system of signification. It is one that he has internalised to such an extent that it influences not only his thinking, and his ways of talking about HIV and himself, but also the way he sees his body. Thus while cultural constructions of HIV have moved on considerably, John has not.

John's experience, as particular as it may be, tells us something about positive lives generally, but in some ways it is very basic. To communicate with other people, an individual has to use a form that will be understood. While illness can be a very private experience, language which speaks about it has to be shared. What John's view of HIV shows clearly is that one often has to draw on existing resources. Certainly this offers some choices. Further, while it is possible to forge some new ways of speaking and writing, this will usually take the discourses already circulating as a necessary departure point.

This interview took place as part of a broader investigation into HIV and quality of life. Respondents in the UK were recruited through some local HIV non-government organisations (NGOs), but by far the majority (including John) contacted me after I placed an advertisement on the web page of *Positive Nation* magazine. Some of these contacts decided they did not actually want to talk. John had made sure I was who I said I was (through some internet and telephone research) and was thus happy to meet with me, as he considered a researcher to be part of the HIV community. John and I initially met away from his home city. Because of the short time available on that occasion, and the failure of recording equipment, we decided to meet again at his house for a whole day. From this, 220 minutes of recorded and transcribed data is used here.[*]

---

[*] Pauses are marked by (.) and line numbers of the original transcript are given: l. indicates a single line, ll. indicates more than one line.

Other matters we discussed will be mentioned, though it will be made clear that these are derived from field notes. The interview was semistructured, covering a number of topics: medication, stigma, relationships, HIV support groups, confidentiality and work. This kind of narrative is not yet routinely circulating[18] as it is from a heterosexual positive man in the UK. I quote John at length in an attempt to give voice to his story. While this is not enough of a reason, it is certainly an important part of work with positive people. The respondents I have spoken to, especially those not involved in the gay community, often remark that there are no representations of 'normal' positive people – that is, people like them.

This particular interaction was unsettling. Even before the extended session I had non-specific reservations about whether I should go. Something about John made me uncomfortable. In retrospect, it is more than likely that he felt the same. To talk to a stranger about the most intimate aspects of one's life and about a condition that you associate with dirt and contagion cannot be easy. Our conversation often became very heated. I repeatedly tried to challenge his vision of himself. I would point out alternative readings and realities that he could enter into. Despite this frustration, I was finally impressed with John's honesty and integrity. For him, there were no alternate readings. The one he had internalised was true. This encounter (as many others in the course of this research) made clear the limits of my understanding. Unless and until HIV happens to my body, it is impossible to say how I would read it.

Framework and structure

The structure of this chapter attempts to mirror the structure of John's extended narrative. In one way, his story can be understood as being structured like a typical claim/denial.[19] The claim is that HIV does not carry stigma, John's denial is that it does. This denial is structured along thematic lines. The themes are realised as episodes in the text.

It is worth being clear about what I mean when I describe a text as 'episodic'. Van Dijk and Kintsch, after suggesting examples of topic change markers, summarise:

> The general strategy, thus, is that if some sentence no longer can be subsumed under a current macroproposition, a new macroproposition will be set up, of which the change markers are the respective partial expressions.[20]

I suggest that to better understand the notion of a 'macroproposition' we understand them as 'themes', related to an overarching 'subject'. I intend 'theme' and 'subject' in this understanding to be drawn from musical rather than from linguistic terminology. Understanding episodic texts in terms of subject and themes accounts for the way in which episodes can recur, or be interrupted or suspended or self-contained.

We can understand the overall purpose of the text as the 'subject' and the premises which support it as 'themes' subordinate to, drawn from or based on the 'subject'. Thus while the individual themes may or may not be related to each other, they all articulate an aspect of the subject or support it in some way. An episodic text, then, can be defined as a text which is a series of articulated and developed themes united by a subject.

The subject captures the point of the text. Unlike a subject in musical compositions, however, it may or may not be articulated explicitly. The themes are derived from material in the subject, as they are in music. The episodes of a fugue, for example, 'are nearly always based upon figures in the Subject or Counter-Subject [answer to the Subject], and…often consist of a sequential treatment of such figures'.[21] Further, the subject–counter/subject interaction can also be related to the notion that argument is dialogic in, for example, Ducrot and Anscombre's understanding. If we understand macropropositions in musical terms, it is easier to understand how episodes can recur, be interrupted, and so on. Musical themes can appear, disappear, undergo transposition, inversion, repetition and various other formal manipulations and substantive embellishments. Thus 'the coherence of the whole is created *solely* by the unity of a few things (and motifs) which are developed in variations' in addition to their relationship to the subject.[22]

The analysis of this interview starts from the structure of John's narratives and explores the themes which achieve this. A structural analysis of this interview shows alternation between five themes. I deal with them in the order that they first occurred in the narrative. After these initial entries, John moves back and forth among the themes. Regardless of questions I asked, all accounts were clear instantiations of one the themes.

John starts talking about the artefacts of HIV (medicine and literature) and how he hides them. In the first section, I deal with this in terms of how John understands himself as being seen by others. Essentially, these episodes deal with how he 'covers' (in Goffman's terms[23]) the stigma of being positive. He then moves on to talking about how positive people are represented, and what he is 'supposed' to look like. This is discussed in the second section. The third theme deals with stigma, including who John can disclose to (his 'own' or the 'wise') and why he cannot disclose to the 'other'. The fourth theme is directly related to the third. John is looking for a relationship, but he will only consider positive women. Finally, the fifth theme (which is implicit in the others, and can be understood as the 'subject') examines what John understands as 'normal'. While he works at passing for normal, he knows that he is not.

How would you know him?

I will begin by looking at the way other people might describe John as it is so strikingly different from the way he sees himself as a positive person. He is a professional, working in a large city. Apart from a severe period of AIDS-related illness four years ago, and a period of unemployment following redundancy, he has been working continually since his diagnosis 13 years ago. Herzlich finds that illness is often associated with inactivity and that '[b]eing off work is an institutionalized stopping of activity'.[17] John often states how he has continued to work and any periods of not working are not (except in one case) directly related to illness. In fact, continuing work is central to John's negotiation of 'normality'. He travels often and socialises with friends and colleagues. John is healthy in that he shows no signs of illness. He is also fastidious that anything material connected with HIV is carefully hidden.

The first thing we talked about was medication. Usually the topic of medication in interviews with positive people revolves around the toxicity of the drugs, the side effects that make day-to-day living uncomfortable or impossible. Sometimes medication is the cause of apparent bodily changes, lipodystrophy, for example. John did not talk about any of these things. He talked about how he disposed of empty medication bottles and how to travel with HIV medication. Medication is important to consider because 'up front it's the extent of' [l. 2154] the effect of HIV on John's life. It is one of the few physical 'symptoms' of his serostatus.

> John showed me a bottle containing fifteen days of medication.
> …in 15 days when it's finished what I do is…take the label and every-thing off and I cut it up with scissors and then *[it]* goes in the bin *[inaudible]* the couple of times I have thrown stuff out to do with HIV on it what I do is I get it in a bag I wrap it twice and I don't put it in the bin here I go down to the skip and preferably I'll have some stuff from doing decorating or something and it'll get dumped in with that so there'll be paint or something to put off anyone. *[ll. 5–10]*

I queried whether anyone would look for something like that. He acknowledged that this was 'sort of paranoia' [l. 12]. The routines he has assembled around any-thing with the letters HIV on it have, however, incorporated this 'paranoia' into daily activities.

Strategies around medication also came into play when travelling. The med-ication is 'disguised' [l. 2156] in other packages so that it 'looked innocent' [l. 2157] with 'all the identifying marks' (l. 2166) taken off. It should be borne in mind that medications are unlikely to have 'HIV' stamped on them. Further, to recognise a drug name as being a treatment for HIV requires specialist med-ical knowledge that only a positive person or someone involved in caring for them would have. Goffman notes that strategies like this, which attempt to control information around stigma might include 'what espionage literature calls a "cover"'.[23] Indeed, the reference to spies is apropos as it occurs around other topics in the interview.

The discussion of medication indicates the importance of John presenting a non-HIV face to the world. While HIV is written in his body (and his behaviour), it is not a legible script. If it was clear that he was positive, there would be no point in engaging in the careful disposal and covering of medication. While the medication bottles are destroyed and camouflaged so that they cannot be found accidentally (or if one was actively looking) other material is hoarded.

> …most of the stuff that I've collected over the three years because it's only three years that I even discovered *Positive Nation* magazine exist-ed so basically there's about three years' supply of stuff and it sits up in the attic and it doesn't really get cleared out because there's all this palaver *[laughter]* about making sure that I wouldn't actually be found with it or no one would trace it back to me. *[ll. 12–16]*

Positive Nation is the UK's HIV and sexual health magazine. It is published by the UKC: the UK Coalition of People Living with HIV and AIDS.[24] The material is incriminating. This is clear not only from the strategies that John employs to dis-pose of or hide it, but also from the lexical choices he makes. He 'disguises' the medication so it looks 'innocent'. The direct implication is that in its natural state it would 'incriminate' him somehow. The notion that material could be 'traced back' to him, that he could be 'found with it', suggests again something illegal. This is the kind of discourse someone might use in relation to illegal drugs. The material here, however, is routine, legally procured and prescribed

HIV medication, and *Positive Nation* magazines. The control of his medication can be understood as *adherence* to normality. The lengths that John goes to indicates the power of HIV as a negative identifier in his wider world.

What is he supposed to look like?

The stereotypical face of HIV for many people is still that of the 'AIDS victim'. I use the term here deliberately to highlight the way in which the mass media, particularly in the late 1980s and early 1990s, portrayed HIV. John comments on the difficulty of orienting to HIV when all that is given is a 'false' view of the illness.

> ...and the ones *[positive people]* who you know bloody Princess Diana goes and visits somewhere and lo and behold there's these mobile skeletons and they have about two months left to live and she holds the hand and makes front page news and you think well hang on I'm not looking like a skeleton yet. *[ll. 86–8]*

The only positive people that many people have seen are those dying of AIDS rather than those living with HIV.[25] John is certainly in the latter category, even though he, like many positive people, has been hospitalised with a CD4 count of zero,[*] AIDS-related illnesses and a bleak prognosis.

Further, the 'yet' signals that he sees this state as inevitable. He says of this period, 'I can never work out quite how near to being dead I was' [ll. 2217–8]. Crimp's analysis in the early 1990s finds that even the person dying of AIDS is not openly shown.

> For the most part, though, they are not seen, or only partially seen, for these are portraits of the ashamed and dying.[26]

He goes on:

> Most often they appear like terrorists, drug kingpins, and child molesters, in shadowy silhouette, backlit with light from their hospital room windows.[26]

In such portraits, if they are less 'ashamed' it is because they are 'innocent'.[26] 'They are so innocent that they can even be shown being comforted, hugged and played with'.[26] This has changed somewhat with the presentation of more heroic figures, such as Tom Hanks's character in the film *Philadelphia*, and the use of characters who happen to be positive, like the character Mark Fowler in the UK soap *Eastenders*.

It is important, however, to note the distinction between the representations that Crimp is dealing with and those in film and television. Crimp's work is commenting on people who are actually positive and how they are represented. Fictional characters are not necessarily bound by the same social and personal constraints as positive people. Conflict, discrimination and acceptance can be scripted in a way that does not always match up with the experience of positive people.

---

[*] CD4 count is a measure of immune system strength as it measures the level of T helper cells in the blood. A CD4 count of zero essentially means that the immune system is not functioning at all.

When John starts talking about HIV and what it signifies, it becomes very clear why he takes such pains to dispose of medication bottles and why he talks about them as though they are incriminating evidence.

Stigma: or what HIV means

I will explain briefly how this mapping relates to the body and HIV's relation to the body and will elaborate further with examples from the transcript. For John, HIV is associated with sex, gayness, transgression, non-normality, death, contagion and stigma. To 'come out' as positive means that these meanings will be mapped onto his person, onto his body. They already are implicitly mapped insofar as this is his understanding of HIV. He quite clearly owns his 'stigma'; essentially this means he has already written these negative meanings of HIV on his own person. It is only possible to be 'out' about his status with those who are of his own 'subculture'. I use the term 'subculture' because John uses it. This is not the subculture of style and behaviour which marks a group out from hegemonic practice (though the status and power relations may be comparable).[27] It is not so much about style as substance – that is, a close relationship with HIV in some way. Further, members of the subculture do not necessarily display their affiliation, it will often be hidden. John uses 'subculture' to refer to his stigma community, those sympathetic others.[23] Sometimes the designation also extends to include the wise, usually those working in the HIV world (nurses, doctors, staff at support groups, and so on).

John has no fear of being discredited in this subculture. Whether this is because they read his positive body differently or because they have no privileged position of 'normality' to judge him, is not clear: but whose words are these written on his body? In part, they come from established myths about HIV; that you have to be homosexual, an intravenous drug user (IVDU), or somehow deviant and immoral to get it. They also come from John's experience of the positive world; one which for many years was largely mediated and obtained from the mass media. I suggest this lack of alternate experiences makes resistant readings of negative representations extremely difficult. In turn this makes alternative narratives becoming public very difficult.

What does seem clear, however, is the physicality of the stigma.[28] Goffman writes:

> ...the Greeks, who were apparently strong on visual aids, originated the term *stigma* to refer to bodily signs designed to expose something unusual and bad about the moral status of the signifier. The signs were cut or burnt into the body and advertised that the bearer was a slave, a criminal, or a traitor – a blemished person, ritually polluted to be avoided, especially in public places.[23]

Goffman notes that the root of stigma is usually detectable. One might miss or cover the implications of the stigma, or even miss or cover the stigma itself, but it is primarily rooted in the physical. HIV is not, however, written on the body in a legible way. Unless one has access to blood and ELISA tests and the like, the HIV is invisible, but the experience of stigma is physical. Because John wants his 'actual social identity' to be constantly hidden among normals (that is, he wants to pass as normal) he is always discreditable.[23]

Thus the 'real' body is kept to the positive world; positive status is only disclosed to others of positive status and those in the field. He can only talk about this 'real' body in a limited space. Body as origin of projection of self in the world can be manipulated such that one appears to be 'normal'. One is not, however, 'normal' because one is positive. I hasten to add that this is not my view. I am only trying to map, and make sense of, what John related to me. He was adamant that I could not understand what it was like to be positive and refused my attempts to 'normalise' or perhaps 'randomise' the fact that he is positive (in that I argued it could happen to anyone). It is also important to note that John reproduces readings of HIV that were in circulation in the late 1980s when he was diagnosed. It seems to me that the point of his diagnosis and the isolation he experienced for the next eight years (during which time he disclosed to no one and did not even meet another positive person) are central to his own lexicon of HIV.

The stigma is difficult to unpack logically. Certainly some of it has to do with the association of HIV with homosexuals. This came up more than once (in fact a dozen times) in the interview, especially in relation to the effects of disclosure. In the following, we also see the association of Black Africans with HIV.

> R: You never considered telling your family?
> J: No no no chance it's just that on the list of people to tell your family would be the lowest on the list you were gonna tell one one one of the reasons was and still is to a certain extent was that the family might think you're gay and I mean I I I mean that's still an issue now but it was certainly a big issue back when it was a gay plague I mean now it's not quite so bad because there's a lot more heteros who are positive and and a lot more black and no one's gonna think of you're black because I'm not but being gay is nothing to do with the colour of your skin so again from a hetero guy's point of view it's like *[inaudible]* if you're down the pub or whatever and you want to insult someone you call them a poof and particularly in the early 90s it was because there weren't that many black Africans coming to the UK with it it was very much a it was gay plague. And the last thing on earth on top of all the other insults would be people thinking I was gay
> R: and especially your family thinking you were gay
> J: Precisely. *[ll. 122–135]*
> *[R refers to myself; J to John.]*

> The perceived melding of AIDS and homosexuality results in the two concepts being stored together in the same cognitive schema in an individual's mind... Regardless of whether homosexual individuals have contracted AIDS *[sic]*, homosexuality is associated with AIDS and vice versa.[29]

There appear to be a limited number of readings of positive status. In fact, here we are presented with what John sees as the two options. First, HIV means one is black. He notes that this is impossible. There is no way this could be written on or read from his white body. The second option, however, gayness, could be because 'being gay is nothing to do with the colour of your skin'. Being HIV positive might signify gayness. He goes on to say that he does not 'know which would be worse, telling them [his parents] I was positive or telling them I was gay' [ll. 140–1]. For John, the two seem to be synonymous in terms of negativity if nothing else.

Disclosing HIV status has been likened to coming out as homosexual.[30] While there is a parallel in the sense that coming out as either gay or positive places one in a minority, it is difficult to extend the analogy. Certainly there are some people who regard homosexuality as an illness. At least in the West, however, being gay is most often understood as being innate. Being gay is not a health state and certainly not a terminal illness. It seems to me that the issues of mortality and stigma that HIV currently evokes, as well as placing one in yet another minority, mean that comparing the two occasions of disclosure can only go so far. That is not to say that HIV disclosure does not resemble 'coming out' as gay in some social settings, especially in the past when scripts for such moments were not in circulation, legal sanctions were in place and gay communities were not as out as they are now.

John's reluctance to disclose his HIV status for fear of being labelled gay might also be read by some as repression of his own homosexuality. Having spent so much time with him I find this difficult to accept. While John would certainly be considered 'homophobic' by many, his unwillingness to be associated with homosexuality is more about him wanting to be 'normal'. I am reluctant to provide great detail about John's upbringing. Perhaps it is enough to say that he comes from a very religious family which has high social standing and visibility in its community. Further, the part of the country in which he grew up is not one in which deviations from masculine norms of any sort are easily accepted. The culture in which John grew up was one that, 'if you're down the pub or whatever and you want to insult someone you call them a poof'.

The concept of the 'gay plague' is an old one. The residue of discourse past is still present and active. Treichler writes: 'Whatever else it may be, AIDS is a story, or multiple stories, read to a surprising extent from a text that does not exist: the body of the male homosexual. It is a text people so want – need – to read that they have gone so far as to write it themselves'.[11] It is clear that homosexuals and intravenous drug users are not considered to be normal in John's view. Whether homosexuals or intravenous drug users (IVDU) are positive or not is immaterial – for John they are not 'normal' people whatever their status. Certainly he does not consider himself normal, his positive status precludes this. However, he carefully segments different kinds of non-normality.

His own 'story' about how he became positive is credible, he argues, and does not relate to homosexuality.

> I have travelled a lot and I've been out to *[another country]* several times the story does stand up well actually it was getting up to no good in *[this other country]* you know so the there it's a risk at all, the icing on the cake of disaster is telling them you've got HIV and the suspicion must be gay must be bisexual whatever I mean it's just not on. *[ll. 144–8]*

While the story 'does stand up', John's understanding of disclosure is that an immediate mapping of gayness or bisexuality would occur and that is 'just not on'. If John is right about the implications of being positive (one must be Black, an IVDU, homosexual or bisexual) there is no reason why this should not happen, as homosexuality is not visible. The credible story of John's infection is not one he wants to tell normal people.

What develops in this train of conversation with John is that stigma comes also from the communicability and incurability of HIV. John sees the fact that the primary mode of transmission is sexual as the root of the stigma.

> I think the only time I'd ever actually tell anyone in fact I'd probably write a book about the whole happy saga, is if they found a cure. Because when it no longer affects anyone else it will cease to be a a a source of of ah stigma *[ll. 153–5]. […]* The big problem with HIV and AIDS as a as an issue is the fact you can pass it on and not only can you pass it on you can you pass it on primarily through sexual contact and that that's why you know if you're wondering why it's a big bloody issue that's why. *[ll. 159–61]*

Sexually transmitted diseases, even if curable, 'are regarded as not the best diseases to have' [l. 173]. He cites the stricter confidentiality of genitourinary medicine clinics (GUM clinics) as a warrant for this. He then draws a parallel between disclosing any other sexually transmitted infection (STI) to family or friends with his decision not to disclose his HIV status.

> I mean if I had gonorrhoea would I tell my parents well don't be bloody stupid it's the last thing you're gonna tell your parents so when so I think I've got HIV which is a sexually transmitted disease or you're gay or I'm an injecting drug user well *[snort]* you know who's the last people you tell well that's your parents and the standard that telling your family is taken to be a good idea with HIV if I had gonorrhoea it wouldn't be a good idea so why is it a good idea with the HIV? *[ll. 175–80]*

Again, the sexual transmission is only part of the problem. The suspicion of homosexuality and drug use figure again here. Other STIs are not equivalent to HIV. Historically speaking, Clark notes that these were 'in the Victorian age regarded as "venial", or forgivable, sins of passion'.[31] HIV is not; it is a sin of deviance.

That John is not gay does not preclude his feeling like a 'plague dog' [l. 1668]. In some untaped remarks he told me that disclosing his HIV status was tantamount to saying one was a paedophile. He refers several times in the taped interview to an exchange he had with another heterosexual positive man.

> …he said he felt dirty and I felt that was probably the best description of what it's like to have it (.) and and and it's always stuck with me he said I feel dirty ever since I had that diagnosis and again the weird thing about it is I feel the same but no one else can see that I feel dirty you know you know I haven't changed colour my hair hasn't fallen out nothing's changed visually but yeah I mean it's just that carrying this thing around that you the other problem is you don't want to give it to anyone else (.) and that becomes really restricting. *[l. 208–13]*

Here the physical and mental aspects of (self-)stigma are captured by feeling 'dirty' and result in 'restriction' from 'carrying this thing around'. This captures the sense of contamination, uncleanliness and moral transgression. Explicitly stating that nothing has 'changed visually' signals that the feeling is nevertheless visceral; that one might have expected physical changes. Clearly he feels polluted.[32] Certainly, following Douglas, he is also in an anomalous position in that he is trying to be 'normal' and yet constantly aware of the fact that he is not. John does not fit into the categories that he is willing to recognise in society.

He says almost the same thing later in the interview, stating again that there have been no physical changes that are visible. Here, he acknowledges the 'irrationality' of his feeling dirty:

> ...it is summed up I feel dirty (.) I feel and again it's kind of because I don't look any different because I don't look like I've got HIV I don't look like a victim or anything I don't act like a victim (.) there's this weird thing that I I I carry it and it's my it's my stigma it's not your stigma or anyone else's it's mine and that that's probably the worst thing and you know people who I've said that to before say well why don't you get rid of it (.) for me the whole AIDS thing would collapse like a pack of cards the moment we get a cure (.) when there's a cure you know I will cease to be a danger to anyone else and even anyone else who did get it for whatever reason (.) there wouldn't be an issue cause you'd take a few antibiotics and a magic treatment potion whatever. *[ll. 1612–21]*

It is apparent here too that the dirt is contagious.*

Who do you love?

> The body...has become...a text to be read, written or rewritten by 'body-experts', be they doctors, beauticians, sports instructors or lovers.[33]

For most positive people relationships highlight the difficulties of living with HIV. In fact, it would be fair to say that in this interview (and many others) close to half the time (if not more) is spent talking about the difficulties of initiating or conducting relationships. The problem with relationships is that because of transmission, and perhaps also because of disclosure, John only considers positive women. This certainly removes some of the problem of when to disclose in a new relationship.[23] In the following, however, the possibility of transmission and stigma in general are backgrounded. The reasons why John does not feel like he could have relationships with negative females is not raised as such. They are presupposed here:

> ...because if you felt you could have relationships with negative females then relationships wouldn't be an issue relationships are an issue because of the whole actual number of people who can have a relationship is measurable in the few hundreds. *[ll. 1484–7]*

The scarcity of women is a concern as it minimises 'chances':

> ...see the big deal for for for for me and anyone who's positive is that chances like this don't come up every week...for me it's a case of, if I don't get on with this girl...when's the next one I'm gonna meet? *[ll. 1024–30]*

John contrasts this with the case of an 'average guy' who would have a far easier time of it. The requirements for John are more difficult. Not only does a potential partner have to be positive, she has to be 'carrying on as normal as well'. [l. 1022]

---

* 'Dirty' is also exactly the term John uses when talking about homosexuals; 'they're [homosexual] dirty buggers' [l. 167], 'you don't want those dirty buggers near us'. [l. 171]

I will return to this concept of 'normality' presently. It is worth noting, however, how John sees confidentiality as working against some of the interests of positive people. In a way, the confidentiality maintained in a GUM clinic is extended to most of the HIV sector involving positive people. Essentially it means that sometimes trying to live in the HIV world is like living in a GUM clinic in terms of confidentiality. While this makes the space safe, it is still a restricted space. This means that trying to meet potential partners in the HIV world is not always straightforward:

> I mean I can't remember what film it was it was *Platoon* or something like that, the first casualty of war is the truth, well I sort of think with HIV, the first casualty of HIV is your friendships and relationships because everyone has the same reaction and they all start drawing back *[pause]. [ll. 213–16]*

None of John's friends know that he is positive, so this 'drawing back' cannot be directly experiential. In relationships, because of physical and emotional intimacy, HIV has to be negotiated in some way. Only considering positive women is part of this negotiation. It removes the possibility of being discredited, as the other person is in the same situation. The 'drawing back' that John talks about echoes in its physical and emotional dimensions his feeling of dirtiness and consequent isolation.

This particular discussion about relationships brought to mind Winterson's novel, *Written on the Body*. Appropriately for discussion here, the narrator's lover has cancer. It has not manifested symptoms. The narrator (whose gender is never revealed) searches for information about bodies with cancer in order to understand the lover she has already abandoned (to the lover's husband's care – a research oncologist). At the start of the novel, the narrator muses:

> Why is it that the most unoriginal thing we can say to one another is still the thing we long to hear? 'I love you' is always a quotation.[34]

John only reveals his real body to positive women; it is only here that he can hope to say and hear 'I love you'. The writing on his body, his feelings of contagion and dirtiness, can perhaps only be read by positive women if there is to be a chance to hear the three word quotation:

> Written on the body is a secret code only visible in certain lights; the accumulations of a lifetime gather there…I like to keep my body rolled up away from prying eyes. Never unfold too much, tell the whole story.[34]

The body can only be unrolled in the presence of someone who can stay still while hearing the whole story. Someone who will not draw back.[29]

Talking and bodies

Talking itself is an embodied act. Gwyn writes: 'voice is the explicit manifestation of the embodied nature of illness'.[4] In terms of 'hidden-ness' it is pertinent that John did not speak to anyone (except physicians, and even then only after an acute period of illness in year eight; before this there was no treatment at all) about his HIV for 11 years:

> partly it was frustrating not being able to talk about it but one of the reasons I couldn't talk about it I mean I knew there must be other

> heterosexuals in the UK with it uhm but I couldn't couldn't work out
> who the hell are they and it's almost like you're a spy and you're in
> the KGB and you're in the UK but you don't know who the other
> bloody KGB agents are. *[ll. 80–3]*

This association with spies and espionage has already briefly been mentioned. It
is perhaps not surprising that Treichler, following Haraway, also finds these
metaphors in scientific accounts of modern immunology.[11]

This silence is impossible to interpret in some ways. It is only when John started to speak about being positive (though in a limited context) that the silence
became at all visible. In relation to communicative silence, which is visible,
Sobkowiak writes:

> Silence must be ranked as the overall least formally complex commu-
> nicative entity. Indeed, except for size (duration), it has no formal
> exponents: no segments, no morphemes, no words to go by, just noth-
> ing (hesitation markers and audible breath-taking do not code CS
> [communicative silence], of course). By this token, then, CS should be
> regarded as (formally) unmarked compared to speech. Similarly,
> although nobody would deny that CS carries content, it would prob-
> ably be agreed that in terms of content complexity CS is indeed
> unmarked relative to speech.[35]

In fact, the limited sphere in which John discloses, and the nature of this space
in terms of confidentiality, means that silence is maintained. His silence, when
uncovered, does express the negative features that Jensen associates with silence:
separation, wounding, concealment and censorship, and dissent/disfavour.
Jensen identifies one more feature, inactivity.[36] The positive corollary of this is
work and thoughtfulness which captures the activities that John pursues in his
effort to be seen as normal. He does not want his silence to be noticed or interpreted. John's silence is not intended or constructed to be communicative.

One can also read John's silence and 'frustration' in a very physical and sexual way. While John could not talk about it because he could not identify someone else appropriate to talk about it to, he felt he could not engage in any kind
of dating or relationship activity. In fact, his first 'relationship' mainly consisted
in talking through his 11 years of silence. This woman 'had this download of all
my frustrations of 11 years of being positive and all the rest of it' [ll. 660–1].
Talking about being positive is a *physical* release. John likens the burden of not
talking about HIV to being in a pressure cooker.

What is normal?

Returning to the start in as far as returning to the body, appearances and deception,
I now try and map John's disjuncture between the normal and the non-normal.
Normal people do not have HIV. What is more, normal people do not *get* HIV:

> I don't understand that thing anyone could have got it whatever (.) if
> I hadn't gone shagging in *[another country]* I wouldn't have it end of
> debate but you know gay guys, if you weren't gay you wouldn't have
> it, drug users if you weren't in sticking bloody needles in your self you
> wouldn't have it (.) Normal people how would I define normal, people

who happily married and are faithful don't do drugs and all the rest of
it they don't get HIV (.) you know so one of the reasons I'm not too
happy about the whole thing is that I I would have liked to be in the
normal group but I know I'm not and I know I'm not because of my
behaviour. *[ll. 1458–65]*

John 'would have liked to be in the normal group' but he is not. As alluded to, his
understanding of what 'normal people' think of HIV is taken from discourses
around HIV at the time of diagnosis, and also from his own stance before his diagnosis. The experience of not being normal is the root of stigma, as Goffman notes.[23]

I mean one of the oddities of having HIV is that if I was negative I'd
be the first person to say ship them off to a desert island and leave
them to bloody rot. *[ll. 1453–4]*

While John has to be said at one level to author his own stigma, it is very clear
that he feels there is no other option. By this I mean it seems clear that he hears
other voices writing the script of HIV; but the voices of the other are also his
voice. Indeed, his congruence is remarkable.
Using an inclusive pronoun he says:

We'll never be bloody open minded about it and least of all because
the people who have got it don't feel open minded about it. *[ll. 1605–7]*

The first 'we' refers to 'the general population'. John includes himself in this 'we'
as well as in 'the people who have got it'. This is a vicious circle. When one is in
the (non-normal) subgroup of positive people, though projecting an image of
normality, the only representations that the normal group will see are AIDS vic-
tims. Positive people are invisible to 'normal' people and to each other. Positive
heterosexuals are particularly invisible; as John notes, it is like being 'in the
KGB...but you don't know who the other bloody KGB agents are' [ll. 81–3].
John's resistance to an alternative reading of his serostatus at this level and his
alignment with the 'general population' indicates the power of the narratives and
myths that are still in circulation about HIV. The cultivation of a 'normal' face can
be theorised with respect to Foucault and his prioritising of the body as a site of
'unique disciplinary power'.[4,37]
Normality is perhaps the central issue for John. While he does not consider
himself to be in the normal group, he acts as though he is. To begin with, he
claims that it is not an act:

...it was just kind of bizarre because it was having this one thing that
you just couldn't talk to absolutely anyone at all about uhm and really I I think it was having to keep keep up the, cause it wasn't really a
pretence because I did everything as normal anyway. *[ll. 77–9]*

While he was 'doing' everything as normal anyway, things were not 'being' normal. Otherwise there would be no 'gulf', there would be nothing 'bizarre' and
there would not be 'this one thing that you just couldn't talk' about. As noted, certain people are sought out for relationships because of similarities in this respect:

...they're *[white women]* a bit like me because they tend to have this
thing that everything's normal on the surface but below it's not normal

and the bit that isn't normal is the fact that they find relationships difficult. *[ll. 259–61]*

Again:

...yeah even though work wise and everything else it kinda looks normal (.) it never has been not at an emotional and personal level. *[ll. 2281–3]*

The craving for normality is a desire to be in that normal group, subject to the same things as everyone else:

I spose the holy grail probably isn't the the the girlfriend in itself it's getting back to being normal I think that's where the cure becomes the critical thing because that means I'm as normal as anyone else (.) and yeah if that means I get run over by a bus and if I then get married get married and have kids get divorced that's bloody normal because everyone gets married and has kids and gets divorced that's what people do (.) and that means I'm back in normality and it's that it's the it's the feeling an outsider which is odd because no one else knows (.) I mean you're one of the few peo you know *[friend's name]* knows, people in GUM clinic know and a few people in the support groups know and that's it (.) and again most of the people I've mentioned are in my subculture anyway (.) *[ll. 2305–13]*

This description of 'normal' is eerily like a passage from an American government information pamphlet, *America Responds to AIDS*:

Married people who are uninfected, faithful and don't shoot drugs are not at risk.[38]

These are almost exactly John's own words [ll. 1458–65]. People in the subculture include positive people, anyone involved in positive support groups, people involved in medical care and those working in some other capacity in the field – for example, as researchers. These can perhaps be called collectively 'wise', along Goffman's lines.[23] What is essential is that people in the subculture do not have a privileged position from which to read John's stigma: because they chose not to take one, or because they are positive. He spoke about this in relation to his position vis-à-vis other positive people:

...and that's why when it comes to me going to support groups well frankly any poncey ideas that I'm better than anyone else (.) they definitely fall away cause actually (.) ... (.) you get it yeah you get it as a result of your own behaviour and I got it from my behaviour it puts me in the same category as the rest of them *[laughter]* so tough shit. *[ll. 1465–70]*

But generally, normal equals negative. When I queried John about 'normal women' he responded:

...well I tend to use normal and negative interchangeably. *[l. 826]*

The support groups provide a 'back place'[23] where disclosure is not required because presence implies positive status, but where issues surrounding HIV can be freely discussed.

Goffman argues that the stigmatised person is not completely accepted by 'normals' and should not expect to be. S/he is part of 'the wider group' but also different 'and…it would be foolish to deny this difference'.[23] The standards which define 'normal' also define (in opposition) John's stigma. Ironically, if he did not so ardently wish to be in that normal group, one would expect his stigma to be less acute; he would not be subject (and subjecting himself) to that discourse. Another difficulty is that it is completely possible for John to pass as normal in most spheres of life. Yet he knows that he is an alien in a normal world. 'The painfulness, then, of sudden stigmatization can come not from the individual's confusion about his identity, but from his knowing too well what he has become' and what he never can become.[23]

Conclusion

Illnesses mean something. Even if the symptoms are not acute, indeed even if they are quiescent. My attempts to interrogate the meaning that John attributes to HIV did not lessen his stigma. It is possible he found my attempts even more alienating as our views were so incommensurable. Perhaps the problem is not what illnesses mean as much as what happens because of such meaning. The gaze that John apprehends as seeing him means that he works toward normality. His body, his silence and his covering strategies are part of this work.

Despite hearing Sontag's call to reject metaphors of illness,[39] Brody argues:

> The major point is that 'to give disease meaning' is not something we can choose to do or not to do. We are inevitably involved in the business of attributing meaning to illness whenever we tell stories about such people or even if we engage in merely medical diagnosis.[40]

Perhaps, however, what the two mean by 'meaning' is not quite the same. Brody appears to be dealing with a more individualised meaning, while Sontag rejects the automatic, routine metaphors and stereotypes that attach to conditions.

Both are right. In the case of John, encouraging him to 'see' or 'understand' that his illness is not stigmatised completely ignores his own experience. It was also, at least for me, impossible. His primary desire is to be normal but for him this is impossible. He can, however, project normality while knowing all the while that this is subterfuge. His requirements are simple: to live as normal a life as possible. While confidentiality, counselling and antiretrovirals are all considered acceptable demands for positive people to make, John's experience at least shows us that some services (such as dating introductions) are not. More importantly, the only stories that John relates to and finds meaning in are those of other positive people exchanged personally. These stories are contraband.*

Either they are not circulated or they are detached completely from their speaker.

Narratives have the power to surprise us, and, if we let them, to experience states that are not ours. Narratives are our way of communing with the other. They allow us access to and experience of our own bodies and illnesses and those

---

* Though the Positive Speakers' initiative, active in many parts of the world, attempts to redress this.

of others. The tool of narrative shows things that blood tests and microscopes cannot. The human technology of narrative offers vistas and possibilities for action and interaction which differ from and complement the medical construction of the body.

References

1 Foucault M (1973) *The Birth of the Clinic: an archaeology of medical perception* [trans Sheridan AM]. Routledge, London.
2 Frank AW (1991) *At the Will of the Body: reflections on illness.* Houghton Mifflin, Boston.
3 Crimp D (1988) *AIDS*: *cultural analysis/cultural activism.* October Books, Cambridge, MA.
4 Gwyn R (2002) *Communicating Health and Illness.* Sage, London.
5 Feyerabend P (1975) *Against Method: outline of an anarchistic theory of knowledge.* NLB, London.
6 Feyerabend P (1987) *Farewell to Reason.* Verso, London.
7 MacCormac ER (1976) *Metaphor and Myth in Science and Religion.* Duke University Press, Durham, NC.
8 Nash C (1990) *Narrative in Culture: the use of storytelling in the sciences, philosophy and literature.* Routledge, London.
9 Rorty R (1987) Science as solidarity. In: JS Nelson, M Allan and DN McCloskey (eds). *The Rhetoric of the Human Sciences: language and argument in scholarship and public affairs.* University of Wisconsin Press, Wisconsin.
10 Patton C (1990) *Inventing AIDS.* Routledge, New York.
11 Treichler PA (1988) AIDS, homophobia and biomedical discourse: an epidemic of signification. In: D Crimp (ed). *AIDS*: *cultural analysis/cultural activism.* October Books, Cambridge, MA
12 Turner BA (1984) *The Body and Society.* Basil Blackwell, New York.
13 Lacan J (1978) *The Four Fundamental Concepts of Psychoanalysis* [trans Sheridan A]. WW Norton, New York.
14 www.aegis.com/pubs/Cdc_Fact_Sheets/1994/CDC94016.html (accessed 17 May 2005).
15 Joughin JJ (1991) Whose crisis? AIDS/plague and the subject of history. In: F Baker, P Hulme and M Iverson (eds). *Uses of History: Marxism, postmodernism and the Renaissance.* Manchester University Press, Manchester.
16 Navarre M (1988) Fighting the victim label. In: D Crimp (ed). *AIDS: cultural analysis/cultural activism.* October Books, Cambridge, MA.
17 Herzlich C (1973) *Health and Illness: a social psychological analysis* [trans Graham D]. Academic Press, London.
18 Couser GT (1997) *Recovering Bodies: illness, disability and life writing.* University of Wisconsin Press, Wisconsin.
19 Hoey M (1994) Signalling in discourse: a functional analysis of a common discourse pattern in written and spoken English. In: M Coulthard (ed). *Advances in Written Text Analysis.* Routledge, London.
20 Van Dijk TA and Kintsch W (1983) *Strategies of Discourse Comprehension.* Academic Press, New York.
21 MacPherson S (1915) *Form in Music.* Joseph Williams, London.
22 Kundera M (1988) *The Art of the Novel.* Faber and Faber, London.
23 Goffman E (1990) *Stigma: notes on the management of spoiled identity.* Penguin, Harmondsworth.
24 www.positivenation.co.uk (accessed 17 May 2005).
25 Crystal S and Jackson M (1992) Health care and the social construction of AIDS: the impact of disease definitions. In: J Huber and BE Schneider (eds). *The Social Context of AIDS.* Sage, London.

26 Crimp D (1992) Portraits of people with AIDS. In: L Grossberg, C Nelson and P Treichler (eds). *Cultural Studies*. Routledge, London.

27 Hebdige D (1979) *Subculture: the meaning of style*. Methuen, London.

28 Brandt AM (1988) AIDS: from social history to social policy. In: E Fee and DM Fox (eds). *AIDS: the burdens of history*. University of California Press, Berkeley.

29 Le Poire BA, Hiroshi O and Hajek C (1997) Self disclosure responses to stigmatizing disclosures: communicating with gays and potentially HIV+ individuals. *Journal of Language and Social Psychology*. **16**: 159–90.

30 D'Cruz P (2003) *In Sickness and in Health*. Stree, Calcutta.

31 Clark KA (1999) Pink water: the archetype of blood and the pool of infinite contagion. In: WN Elwood (ed). *Power in the Blood: a handbook on AIDS. Politics and communication*. Lawrence Erlbaum, London.

32 Douglas M (1966) *Purity and Danger*. Routledge, London.

33 Fox N (1993) *Postmodernism, Sociology and Health*. Open University Press, Buckingham.

34 Winterson J (1992) *Written on the Body*. Cape, London.

35 Sobkowiak W (1997) Silence and markedness theory. In: A Jaworski (ed). *Silence: interdisciplinary perspectives*. Mouton de Gruyter, Berlin.

36 Jaworski A (1997) Aesthetic, communicative and political silences in Laurie Anderson's performance art. *Silence: interdisciplinary perspectives*. Mouton de Gruyter.

37 Frank AW (1995) *The Wounded Storyteller*. University of Chicago Press, Chicago.

38 WAUDAG (University of Washington Discourse Analysis Group) (1989) Resisting the public discourse of AIDS. *Textual Pract*. **3**: 388–96.

39 Sontag S (1991) *Illness as Metaphor and AIDS and its Metaphors*. Penguin, Harmondsworth.

40 Brody H (1987) *Stories of Sickness*. Yale University Press, New Haven.

Chapter 4

When narratives matter: men, sport, and spinal cord injury

Andrew C Sparkes and Brett M Smith

Imagine having a life story that in the telling involves being a fit, able-bodied, young man with a disciplined and dominating body as described by Frank[1] who loves playing sport, and rugby union football in particular.*

Also imagine a life story in which, over the years, the central themes have revolved around the development of a strong athletic identity and a sense of self based on a performing body.[2]

Now imagine this:

> In the first half *[of the rugby match]*, the centre shoulder charged me out off the pitch. It was a challenge really. I landed heavily on my left shoulder, it hurt like hell but I was only out on the wing anyway. It was an important game, we had no replacements so I struggled on until half time and had a bit of a rub down. I thought, 'Well I can manage.' But, at the time when he shoulder charged me out, I got up and thought, 'All right sunshine, we've got another half to go yet.'

> In the second half, we turned up the pressure. It must have been about five or 10 minutes to go until the end of the match *[silence for eight seconds]*. We were winning, my shoulder was still giving me gyp, so I could have come off really. But, it was pay back time and I won't forget it. I remember they were coming at us, they were in their own half, there was I on the wing and he *[the centre]* was outside. I should have been marking my own wing but for some reason I decided it was time to get him back. So I came inside, which I shouldn't have, I don't know why, I was never a dirty player. I don't know why, but we were both running at quite a speed towards each other and for some reason I was going to take him high, which I never thought I played like that before in all the years. I'd had a few fights yeah, sometimes come off for them, but that's just the way I am – I take the rough with the

---

* The *disciplined body* presents itself as highly controlled and predictable and as lacking desire to engage and commune with other bodies. It is also dissociated from itself and isolated in its own performance even though this performance might be part of a collective institutional activity such as sport. The *dominating body* defines itself by force. It meets the challenge of events, like sport or spinal cord injury (SCI), by trying to beat it. The voice and narrative is dominated not by resignation or an imperative to develop the self, but by anger and frustration. It is also dissociated from itself and lacks desire, but it is dyadic in how it relates to other bodies. Thus, rather than communing with other bodies, it displaces its anger and frustration against its own limits on to others.

smooth... Then, then, *[silence – five seconds]* then as he *[the centre]* got closer and closer, in a very split second I changed my mind, sort of changed my position, just fractionally.

This was in a split second, he dipped his shoulder at the same time as I lowered my position and his shoulder hit me straight on the top of my head. It was a bang against a brick wall really. There was no pain or nothing, just sounded like the crack of a gun going off. And the next minute I was lying on the floor saying: 'Can you put my arms and legs down on the floor.' Strange thing to say, strange thing to feel because my arms and legs felt as if they were raised to the sky and yet it never dawned on me at first that I couldn't feel the rest of my body... It just never dawned on me that maybe I was paralysed... When I had my accident I thought: 'Bloody hell lads, is that happening really?' It's like being struck by lightning... It's difficult to put it into words really.

This is the moment, immortalised in time,[3] when Jamie, a husband, father of three children, crane driver and dedicated rugby player suffered a spinal cord injury (SCI) at the T2 level that propelled him from the world of the able-bodied into the world of the disabled.

The severity of his spinal trauma is such that he now requires artificial life support and breathes using a ventilator. Jamie has no sensation or movement below the neck. Shortly after the SCI, Jamie's wife divorced him. He is currently unemployed, lives in a new bungalow, his children visit him fortnightly, and he has two female care assistants. Concisely, in a turning point moment Jamie's life story changed dramatically. And, even though he states: 'It's difficult to put it into words really', this is exactly what he does as he constructs an autobiographical story post-SCI to make sense of who he was, who he is now, and who he might be in the future.

According to Medved and Brockmeier,[4] autobiographical stories are self-narratives by which we give situation specific answers to the questions: 'Who am I?' and 'What is my life about?' In telling such stories, 'people give meaning to their experiences within the flow and continuously changing contexts of life... All this is done not only in narratives about the past and the present, but also about future times and places'.[4] As these stories of a life are told they operate to provide a structure for our very sense of selfhood and identity.[5] Indeed, for Brockmeier and Carbaugh, 'the self in time – can *only* exist as a narrative construction'.[6]

Personal stories based on remembered experiences, Miller suggests,[7] are an important site for the social construction of self in which facets of self and various identities are projected and maintained over time. For her, selves, like cultures, 'are not so much preserved in stories as they are created, reworked, and revised through participation in everyday narrative practices that are embedded in and responsive to shifting interpersonal conditions'.[7] Therefore, while the individual autobiographical story that is told at any moment in time may seem unique to the teller, it is, in fact a social creation. As Murray[8] reminds us:

> We are born into a culture which has a ready stock of narratives which we appropriate and apply in our everyday social interaction.

In this regard, Somers[9] makes the following observation about the findings from narrative studies:

> Their research is showing us that stories guide action; that people con-
> struct identities (however multiple and changing) by locating them-
> selves or being located within a repertoire of emplotted stories: that
> 'experience' is constituted through narratives; that people make sense
> of what has happened and is happening to them by attempting to
> assemble or in some way to integrate these happenings within one or
> more narratives; and that people are guided to act in certain ways, and
> not others, on the basis of the projections, expectations, and memo-
> ries derived from a multiplicity but ultimately limited repertoire of
> available social, public, and cultural narratives.[9]

Importantly, as the comments made by Jamie earlier reveal, the understanding of one's self in autobiographical time is *embodied*. In talking of the 'body inescapable', for example, Connell[10] notes:

> Bodily experience is often central in memories of our lives, and thus
> our understanding of who and what we are.

Likewise, Watson[11] observes that 'the salience of embodiment can be explained in terms of the relationship that pertains between the body/self and time'. Smith and Watson[12] support these views and point out that the body is a site of autobi-ographical knowledge because memory itself is embodied. For them, 'life narra-tive is a site of embodied knowledge because autobiographical narrators are embodied subjects. Life narrative inextricably links memory, subjectivity, and the materiality of the body.'

What, however, does all this mean for men like Jamie, and what does all this mean for how we understand how narrative works in the lives of people? To explore these issues, we will draw on data generated from a life history study of a small group of men (n=14) who have suffered SCI and become disabled through playing the contact sport of rugby football union.

The methodological and ethical principles informing this study and our work with these men has been described in detail elsewhere in Smith and Sparkes;[13,14,15] Sparkes;[2,16,17] and Sparkes and Smith.[18,19] Suffice it to say here that contact was made with participants via an open letter in a newsletter circulated by the English Rugby Football Union's support network for injured players. The participants then contacted us and engaged in a series of confidential, tape-recorded interviews that explored their life histories pre- and post-SCI. At the first interview the ethical prin-ciples informing the research were discussed with each participant – for example, participants were told they could withdraw from the interview or the study at any time without having to give any reason, that pseudonyms would be used and place names changed to preserve anonymity.

By providing an overview of our findings to date, we seek to illustrate the ways in which certain metaphors, notions of time and certain kinds of hope congre-gate and coalesce within three specific narrative types available to these men within a Western cultural repertoire (*see* Table 4.1). These are the restitution, chaos and quest narratives as defined by Frank[1] that operate to shape the indi-vidual experiences of these men following SCI in terms of how they reconstruct body/self relationships over time. By dealing with each of these in turn, we attempt to reveal that narratives *do* matter when people are faced with disruptive and turning point moments in their lives.

Living in restitution

The restitution narrative framed 11 of the men's life stories. According to Frank[1] the plot of this narrative has the basic story line: 'Yesterday I was healthy, today I'm sick, but tomorrow I'll be healthy again.' For the men in our study, this translates as: 'Yesterday I was able-bodied, today I'm disabled, but tomorrow I'll be able-bodied again.' Within the frame of this narrative, sporting or 'war' metaphors were prominent in these self stories.[14] The most common was associated with *a fight to make a comeback*. This is displayed in the following comments by a participant: 'One thing rugby taught me was that you have to *fight* if you are going to get anywhere in life. I've taken this view into how I see disability and myself now. Because, I will walk again and make a *comeback*. I will *fight* to make a *comeback*.' The other men also made links with sporting struggles when talking about their disability experience. Often the issue of fighting and making a comeback were related to the notion of a medical cure for SCI. This is evident in the following comment by one of the participants as he thinks about what he would like for his future:

> A cure. That is what I want, and I do think that I'll make a *comeback* and walk again at some point in time. I won't stop *fighting* until I can do that... If I'm to *fight* this and make a *comeback*, then religion or believing that I can mentally make myself walk again is useless. Medical progress is what I want and need... My attitude, right from my days playing rugby up until now is to *fight* and to never give in. And I do think that giving in is to admit that you'll never walk again or that you won't get some functioning back. So I have to *fight* and try and make a *comeback*, get back my old self, and wait for a cure. And, well, I have to be strong. I could never give up or stop *fighting*, because that again would be like saying that I'm a failure.

Table 4.1 Narrative types and specific characteristics

Narrative	Restitution	Chaos	Quest
Metaphors	Sport/war: for example, fighting, battle and comeback	Choking and darkness and emotional selves are brittle objects	Journey: for example, reborn, distance travelled and difficulties with travelling
Time	Philosophy of the future The past in the future The present in the future The future in the past Waiting Consumed	Empty present The future in the present Static	Reclaimed Fragmented The past in the past The present in the present The future in the future Consumed Ingested
Hope	Concrete	Despair	Transcendent
Type of self	Restored and entrenched	Fragmented	Developing
Type of body	Disciplined	Chaotic	Communicative

In restitution, another prevalent metaphorical characteristic that strongly shaped the participants' senses of self involved the notion of *winning as being cured of disability*. Here typical statements included: 'Spinal injury is a *battle*, a *struggle*… I will *win* and walk again', and 'It's a long *battle*, but *winning*, which means walking again, is my aim and it's how I feel and look at life.' A further recurring metaphorical strand in the men's stories was one where disability and impairment was defined as an *enemy* that must be *beaten*. This is evident in the following comment: 'It's like in sport, disability is an *enemy* that I must *beat*. But of course I can't do it on my own. I need medicine to find a cure to *win*.' Not surprisingly the *body as a battleground* metaphor was also commonly used, for example, as one participant stated: 'The body is the problem, or at least one of the major problems. I feel as though I'm doing *battle* with it, if it's getting out of bed, out of the bath, out of my chair… And, it feels as though it's in a *relentless battle*, one *long battle* going on inside… One long *battle* against the body until medicine finds a cure and I can walk again.'

The metaphors outlined above are connected to how the self in time is experienced within the restitution narrative. As we have described elsewhere,[19] autobiographical time within this narrative structure reverberates with what Crossley[20] terms a *philosophy of the future*. With respect to disability, this is a temporal orientation that embodies a strategy of minimisation insofar as the person is determined not to let SCI 'ruin' the plans they had in the past, or held for the future. People who develop this temporal mode of living also decline to relinquish their routine future orientation, thus refusing to entertain the possibility that they might not walk again. As one of the participants commented:

> My aim now is to focus on the future and the light at the end of the tunnel… I try and think about what the future has in store, look to there, and wait until a cure is found. I don't think that's strange, because that's what I want, and you know, it's not how I want to live, like this… I want to, and will walk again, and not far in the future a cure will be found, and it's only there that I see myself.

Framed by the demands of the restitution narrative for themes relating to the technology of a cure and the restorable body/self, a narrative connection is made to the basic temporal orientation of living in the future. For this participant, however, like those others who tell restitution stories, the future takes on different meanings because of the relationships that exist between it and the past and present in his life story. Thus, as described by Roberts,[21] he experiences, and shifts between, three time tenses connected through the future: the *past in the future*, the *present in the future*, and the *future in the past*.

Making reference to the *present in the future*, for example, the same participant said:

> Well, it's like this. I don't see any use in thinking about the present, my priority is the future…and that is because I see medical advancements being made, even now as we speak.

Later in the same interview, however, he made connections with the time tense of the *past in the future*:

> When I first came home I'd got very little use in my arms, I'm the strongest I've ever been now… In maybe 10 or 15 years time, I will be as good as new.

Finally, talking about a return to the former self, as well as the future in the past while he waits for a cure that will return him to an able-bodied state of being, this participant stated:

> Keeping who I was in the past, keep it in mind is something that I need to do if I am to get myself back. And if, as I believe, disability is a temporary situation for me, then I want my old self back because I liked myself then… It's knowing that a cure will be available which helps me to keep my perspective on time in the future. So I look to the future, knowing that the past will return, and recapturing what I had can only be accomplished through what lies in medical advancements, progress. You see, it's a matter of believing that. I just know those days will come back. But the problem is the waiting. I sit here, I can hardly get up and walk can I *[laughs]*. Well, just waiting, waiting for the future. Just waiting…waiting for the day when I can walk again, be myself.

These comments signal how this individual narrates time in relation to the future and through the time tenses of the *past in the future* and the *future in the past*. They also highlight how defining SCI as temporary fosters a sense of what Charmaz[22] terms *waiting time*. That is, the restitution narrative evokes feelings of boredom and time is lost while waiting for the body/self to be restored by advances in biomedicine. As this participant stated:

> I don't do a lot, boring existence, just existing… But while it can often seem that I have lots of time on my hands, what you have to remember is that doing the simple things that I never gave much thought about when I could walk, simple things like making a cup of tea, now take up a lot of my time and energy.

In this way, waiting time is connected to *consumed time*, which Seymour[3] describes as an active and ongoing process whereby quantifiable time becomes a scarce resource that must be re-embodied and constantly managed in order for the body to remain healthy, to conform to social imperatives and to achieve satisfaction in life's activities. In doing so, time becomes a commodity and large amounts of time debits must be set against the value of the outputs.

For the participants who told restitution narratives, the metaphors and the time tenses used sustain a sense of *concrete hope*.[15] According to Marcel,[23] this kind of hope is oriented to specific or material results. It is similar to the typical definition of hope used in the psychological literature as 'the positive expectation of realising desirable outcomes'.[24] A sense of concrete hope, partly framed by the demands of the restitution narrative is connected to themes relating to the technology of a medical cure and the restorable body/self. An example of this kind of hope is displayed in the following comment of one of the participants:

> So becoming disabled was not what I expected, and when it happened I lost everything. It was, *is*, such a huge crisis and because of it I've lost my life. So, every day I tell myself that I'll walk again. That's what gets me out of bed in the morning. I don't work and don't play sport anymore. So, what do I really have to look forward to? Well, I have hope. It's about every single day hoping that I'll walk again. Which might sound crazy to some people but at least in this miserable existence I have

hope… I look forward to the day when I can get everything back that I had before the accident. Stand, and walk. So, really, the main thing that keeps me going is the hope I'll recover. Hope that medicine will keep progressing and find a cure. Hope that there will be an end to all this.

Hope in restitution narratives, therefore, is linked to concrete outcomes that revolve primarily around the discovery of a 'cure' via medical and technological advancements in the future. The metanarrative of restitution and concrete hope, along with its associated metaphors and specific time tenses helps create and sustain a *restored* self and an *entrenched* self* as described by Charmaz.[25]

These kinds of self are linked to notions of a 'comeback' that returns the individual to a former, more desirable, state of being that he had in the past. As such, the individual becomes locked into his past body/self relationships and ways of being in the world through the belief that he will return to this state. To be ready for this return, the body itself must remain disciplined and adhere to various therapeutic regimes so that its former predictability can be embraced when the opportunity arises.

Living in chaos

According to Frank,[1] *chaos narratives* are the inverse of restitution narratives, since here the plot imagines life never getting better. These stories are chaotic in their absence of narrative order. They are told by a storyteller who inhabits a chaotic body about how life is experienced – that is, without sequence or discernible causality. Not surprisingly, the self in this narrative is fragmented. Jamie, who suffered his SCI at the T2 level, and who described this moment at the beginning of this chapter, was the one participant who adhered to this narrative form. The metaphors he used when describing his experiences include that of *choking*.

> Before the accident I was happy and life was good. The injury and everything that has happened since has *choked* any life and happiness out of me. I have nothing now *[five-second silence]*. Am nothing. That's how it is and how it will be… Each day is another day that life is *choked* out of me. And I feel as though I'm *suffocating [seven-second silence]*. There is no way out. The body is *choking* me. I don't want any more out of my life. It's over.

Another metaphor for life in chaos used by Jamie is connected to the imagery of *solid darkness*. When asked how he felt about his life now, he replied:

> It's over *[15-second silence]*. I feel removed from my life and from the world outside, as if *darkness is closing in on me*. That's how it feels.

---

* *The restored* self is an identity level at which people expect to return to their former lives following SCI. This is viewed as a 'normal' or 'natural' response. The men who desire this identity level thus aim both to reconstruct a similar physical self as before and assume continuity with the self they had before they became disabled. Restoring an *entrenched* self means being wedded to a clear self-conception situated in the past. This self represents patterns of action, conviction and habit built up over the years. These unchanged patterns had been a source of self-respect before they experienced SCI and became disabled, and once science has 'repaired' their broken bodies, resuming these patterns becomes the person's major objective.

Darkness. But *no light shining through*. It's difficult, because this feeling is present all the time. I'm on my own. No one. Separated from the outside world. I just watch the fish *[in the fish tank]*. *Darkness is pressing in on all sides [five-second silence]*. I'm, I don't know…I can't imagine life without *darkness*. My life is in *darkness*.

In describing being plunged into chaos and feelings of disconnection, Jamie spoke of the *emotional self* as a brittle *object*.

I don't really feel anything *[now]* about myself. I was *shattered* by the accident, and everything *crumbled away* from *underneath* me. It's still *crumbling*. I feel myself *crumbling*… Not being able to control the body, the environment around you, are aspects of life that you have to live with. No matter how much you try, the situation isn't going to be changed. My life since the accident has *fallen apart*, and with it all hope crushed *[five-second silence]*. And things are not going to change. My emotions have taken enough and I'm *shattered*. My emotions are *shattered*. I'm *shattered*.

When chaos moves into the foreground of a self-narrative, and the self becomes fragmented or shattered, the past, present and future come under ontological threat. Accordingly, living in chaos results in time being defined as an *empty present*. This temporal orientation, according to Crossley,[20] refers to time experienced as a stream of overpowering events. Accordingly, people do not think about, plan or commit themselves to future possibilities because they are afraid of disappointment. The anxiety associated with such fears means that they fail to commit themselves to various projects and possibilities, and therefore lose all sense of meaning and coherence in their lives. Finally, time caves in.

For Jamie, embodied experiences of time also encompass a *time tense* of the *future in the present*,[22] that is, experiences of time are arranged and placed by 'reading' through a combination of the present and future. Here, a future is storied as existing in the chaos of the present. In doing so, and with no plans and few resources, composing a future becomes more and more difficult. Consequently, the future turns out to be uncertain. At the same time, the future is undesired since it is imagined as more chaos, or even worse. Moreover, narrative wreckage engulfs the present. Jamie feels trapped in the present. The present swells to fill what is left. The past loses its order and a culturally derived sense of being propelled through time erodes.

Life moves on without me, but, then, I just survive. I don't have ambitions or a future. See the kids grow up, but well it's not the same, then, then what?… I don't do anything of importance. Watch television, not a lot I can do. Nothing *[five-second pause]*. Avoid, just existing. Then, well, life has stopped. Just, I don't know. Exist in the present, no tomorrow, nothing. I don't know where my life is going. Then, but, it's difficult because time means nothing now… Not a lot to live for…time is, is distorted. Just nowhere. I don't know where I am.

Jamie's narrative is also framed by a *static* view of life. This view of life, as described by Brockmeier,[26] is a 'state of mnemonic paralysis, overpowered by all experience that, like a psychological black hole, absorbs all possible development, all movement that could lead the autobiographical process away from this all consuming experience'. This unchanging story of life, the stretched quality of static time that engulfs the person in a sea of dimensionless time, is displayed in the following comment:

> I can't really see a future – I can't. Thinking about, if I could, would be just too overwhelming. I just can't… Life has stopped. Time is frozen. Days, weeks, just merge into one. Nothing changes. Then, I don't know *[five-second silence]*. Things take an eternity to do. So you don't try to do anything anymore. That's why I'm stuck in a rut. In my life nothing changes. Nothing.

The metaphors and time tenses that operate within the chaos narrative leave Jamie with little sense of hope. As he stated:

> My life? It's over… I have nothing left to live for. I have no hope of a life. I have nothing. There is no hope for me.

In despair, life is deemed to be meaningless and devoid of purpose:

> I'm useless. Nothing. My condition won't improve. No point anymore. I'm no one now. It's a matter of sitting here alone until I die. Life ended for me the day I broke the neck… Believe it or not, I was big and strong. Now I am nothing. Life moves on, without me. That is how it is. How it will always be. I just survive. No ambitions. Nothing… Sometimes I don't think I can go on. I do. But life won't improve. It can only get worse… There is no hope in my life.

In chaos Jamie feels swept along, without control, by life's fundamental contingency. His comments also reveal that when hope is lost, or absent, and certain metaphors and time tenses shape experience, then the belief emerges that one's life is, for all intents and purposes, finished. According to Freeman,[27] in situations where certain outcomes are anticipated as inevitable, where things cannot be otherwise, individuals may experience what he calls *narrative identity foreclosure*. This involves the premature conviction that one's life story is effectively over. In such instances, Freeman suggests, if one already knows, or *believes* one knows what lies ahead, then one may become convinced there is little value in lasting to the very end. Consequently, one's life may seem a foregone conclusion. The individual in this circumstance might feel that he or she can no longer move creatively into the future.

Living in quest

In contrast to restitution and chaos narratives, *quest* narratives meet suffering head on. They accept impairment and disability and seek to *use* it. As Frank points out,[1] just what is quested for may never be wholly clear, but the quest is defined by the person's belief that something is to be gained from the experience. Two of the men in our study (David and Doug) told this type of story about themselves. As we have noted elsewhere,[14] within a quest narrative journey metaphors are common. The most prevalent metaphor used in this kind of narrative involved the image of being *reborn*. David stated, for example:

> My life has changed since the accident and I'm now on a *journey*. This isn't a tragic *journey* though. No, I've been *reborn*, and have become a better person since becoming disabled.

Likewise Doug commented:

> I'm on a different *journey*, more positive, and have been *reborn*. I'm learning different things as well, and I've come to think that on this *journey*, yes disability can be a shattering experience and a tragedy for some people. But it shouldn't be. Why? Because it's an opportunity to explore yourself and become a better person… Still, that doesn't happen overnight, and people stress the negative side of disability, how tragic it all is. And for me, if people see it like that, then how can they improve? Also, part of being *reborn* and changing into different person…it meant coming to understand that controlling my body and physical functions just isn't possible. I understand that now, and know that it's not perfect, and that on this *journey* my body will reveal its limitations. But I accept that, and I think that if others can accept it, then maybe people's views on disability might be different and we all might be happier and live better lives.

The 'reborn' metaphor suggests that a serious disruption in life's prospects and expectations can offer some people an opportunity to remake themselves. This remaking rejects an overemphasis on bodily predictability in favour of accepting its contingency as part of the fundamental contingency of life. It also rejects the tragedy story line so often associated with becoming disabled. This said, other journey metaphors used by these two men acknowledge that the reconstructing of body/self relationships, and the transcending of one's narrative resources on becoming disabled, is not easy. Thus there was often talk of the *distance travelled* and the *difficulties with travelling* that signalled both the notion of progress and a number of embodied problems that can occur on becoming disabled. As David commented: 'I've *covered a lot of ground*… I've made a lot of *progress*, but there are a lot of *ups* and *downs* on the *journey* I'm on. It isn't easy.' Doug also felt he had '*moved forward* since the accident…come a *long way*, and made a lot of *advancements…progressing*, not only individually, but also in my relationships with other people'. Doug acknowledged, however, that individual and structural problems can occur as part of the journey:

> *Along the way* there are a lot of problems that can *force* me *off* the *track*… I can't take life for granted. For one, I know that there will be a *rocky road ahead* of me at some point and *obstacles* to think about. For now, I have to contend with everyday *barriers* placed by society, and the occasional emotionally bad day, but who knows what the future will bring.

The metanarrative of progress drawn on by these two men highlights how this complex aspect of journeying is not without risks, difficulties, uncertainties and descents. Comments made by them also signal that on journeys people may need to reach out to others in order to be helped by them. As such, the point of their lives is not found in solitude but partly in stories and dialogue – in communication and community – with others. In this scenario, a more communicative relation with the body emerges in which the body's contingency is not defined as a problem but as a source of possibility.

The journey metaphor involving *guides*, common in both David and Doug's stories, also helps draw attention to this idealised type of body and its empowering potential, as well as to the point that the materiality of the body does matter. As David commented:

> People are like *guides*, helping and *guiding* people along their *journey*. So, one really important part of how I've changed has to do with the *advice* people have offered me over the years, especially since most of it wasn't forced… For instance, I've heard a lot of stories about the disability movement and how society, government policies, access, stuff like that contributes to the problems we face as disabled people… The *advice* and *guidance* from some disabled people has also helped me deal with the practical aspects of disability, and learn to understand the limits of what my body can do and cannot do.

As this comment suggests, stories and counternarratives linked with a political narrative and the liberating and empowering potential of the *social model* of disability can play a significant role in teaching people how to interpret their own disability experiences and the experiences of others. They are also one road to restorying the self over time and developing a more communicative body.[1]

Furthermore, within the quest narrative, there is a re-embodiment of time that points toward new opportunities and a chance to remake a life that has passed.[20] One important aspect of this process includes *reclaimed time*. For Seymour,[3] a serious disruption in life's prospects and expectations can offer people an opportunity to remake themselves, in a sense, to reclaim time that has passed. Here, the reality of irrevocable change, the acceptance of contingency as part of the fundamental contingency of life, and the prospect of an unknown future may give immediacy to life that was formerly taken for granted. In this regard, Seymour suggests:

> By repossessing the past a person may abandon or rework an earlier life script: the 'cleaned slate' may enable the person to reconstitute him or herself in a more purposeful manner.[3]

As David commented:

> Now I appreciate time more, know that I won't live forever, and I try and savour the moment. See, it's a journey, and the time aspect is not something that I take for granted now… Certainly I don't see disability as a tragedy… As well as the social and access problem…disability is also about living within the limitations, the functional ones, not thinking that you can beat them… Some people spend all their time trying to do more, but I think you can waste time like that. We all only have so much time and wasting it, throwing yourself into doing more, trying to walk again. I don't know because I don't want to sound negative, each has their own way, but sometimes it's best to accept it, use it, and try and enjoy the moment.

David's notion of reclaimed time draws, in part, on what Brockmeier[26] identifies as the *fragmentary model* of time. This is a timeless model that recognises the unpredictable nature of human life and the complexity of self. The future, for David, is not completely uncontrollable, but simply less amenable to control. Acknowledging this, he recognises and challenges the myth of control in relation to the body that prevails in Western cultures. Rejecting this myth and recognising that the neither the future nor his body can be totally controlled does not lead David to despondency, or a sense of powerlessness. It simply means that contingency is now accepted as part of the fundamental contingency of life, which is influenced by numerous factors, many of them beyond the control of the individual. Here, as Frank suggests,[1] bodily predictability comes to be regarded as exceptional, and contingency comes to be accepted as normative. As David said:

> I take life as it comes. I don't worry about what the future holds, I mean, I can't control it, not totally anyway, what life throws at you...
> So I take each day as it comes, and enjoy the moment.

David's connection to a fragmentary narrative model of autobiographical time also links him to certain types of 'time tenses'.[21] These include the *past in the past*, the *present in the present*, and the *future in the future*. Making reference first to the *past in the past* and then shifting to a time tense of the *future in the future*, David remarked:

> The past is in the past and the future, well, as I say you have to recognise that the future is too far ahead, but you are still moving.

Later in the interview, however, his accounts of disability are embedded within the *present in the present*.

> I live in the present... I do think that if I lived in the past or thought too much about the future, even if that was concerned with a cure, I don't think that's a good strategy. Why? Well, for starters the present is much more fun... But if I did become preoccupied with the future or even the past, then I think that places a limitation on who you can be... For instance, if I was concerned with the future, then I would probably lose sight of the present and who I am, or am becoming. In that sense, I don't think I would develop as a person because, you know, living in the past or future requires you to have a very specific focus and restricts your opportunities to try out different roles, or experiment with who you are. And in the end I probably would not enjoy the present, not like I do now...I mean, at the end of the day, I live for the here and now and don't take notice of the past, what it meant to me.

Such comments not only signal a life lived in the present, but also suggest that an overemphasis on the past or future might, for some people, lead to a situation that restricts their opportunities to engage with other possible or potential identities as they present themselves. For David, memories of being able-bodied are situated in the past, while living as a disabled person occupies the present and helps shape a future. Therefore, time horizons stay close and neither past nor future assumes priority. The present is attended to with a sense of passion, communion and involvement that enables it to feel fully lived and infused with a certain kind of hope.

In contrast to the restitution narrative that incorporates concrete hope, and the despair of chaos, quest stories foster and embrace *transcendent hope*. This kind of hope, as defined by Marcel,[23] is not oriented to achieving a fixed and specific outcome, but instead embraces uncertainty and finitude, celebrating surprise, play, novelty, mystery and openness to change. In this sense, according to Barnard, 'the hopeful person, rather than being defined (or enslaved) by particular wishes, is continually open to the possibility that reality will disclose as yet unknown sources of meaning and value'.[24] An example of this kind of hope is evident in the following comment of Doug's as he reflects on how he feels about life now:

> Right now I feel great about life and myself… I've developed a much more rounded personality and have become a different person, a much better one after the accident I think, with lots of different sides to me… Okay, for a period of time after the accident I was a mess. But now, I don't view disability as a crisis. I'm on a different path, and I think a better, more fulfilling one. So I'm happy… I don't want to go back to my old life. That doesn't mean that I don't have hopes and dreams. I'm still a hopeful person, but it's not about a cure as many people might think… I don't hope for a cure, and, in my view, it's still very unsure whether one will come… So, I don't live with the hope for a cure… My view of hope is more about a hope for a better world… But I don't really know what that will mean because I'm still learning. And I think part of the beauty of life is not knowing what will happen in the future. Life is uncertain. I enjoy this though, and feel that part of life is learning to live and enjoy just how mysterious and beautiful it can be.

As David commented:

> Hope for me now is about having opportunities, living in a better society that respects disabled people and values them, and not feeling tied down to one life plan. Actually, I like the fact that my future isn't clear, and I look forward to continuing developing myself, learning, and having hope that I can enjoy life and live with all the problems and surprises that goes with it.

Clearly, for David and Doug, within a quest narrative, specific metaphors and certain time tenses operate to sustain a transcendent sense of hope that shapes their post-SCI experiences and their identity construction as disabled men. For them, becoming disabled through sport is reframed as a challenge and an opening to other ways of being. David and Doug have developed more communicative bodies, bodies which place the past securely behind them, live in the present, and see the future as a vista of possibilities, and thus a *developing* self, as described by Charmaz,[25] emerges.

Here, rather than simply committing to an outcome tied to a cure, and being locked into specific prior activities and former identities, David and Doug are concerned about the direction of their lives as well as the character of the self they shape along the way. Indeed, the two men commit themselves to growing and developing in the future. By opting for a developing self these men emphasise their ability to reconstruct their sense of self over time, they display openness to change and show a willingness to explore new identities as possibilities emerge.

Summary

In this chapter, we have illustrated the ways in which different types of body/selves, metaphors, notions of time, and certain kinds of hope, congregate and coalesce within the restitution, chaos and quest narratives that shape the individual experiences of 14 men who have become disabled through sport. These three specific narrative types appear to be important dynamos of their life stories, which energise or impose a structure on what can be experienced and expressed in relation to the lives they could lead.

The restitution narrative leads 11 of the men to articulate sporting/war metaphors, a sense of concrete hope, and a set of time tenses directed toward the future. All of which helps create a restored self and a self that is entrenched, wedded to the former disciplined body which was cultivated in an able body and situated in the past. In contrast to the restitution narrative drawn on by the majority of the men, is the chaos story told by Jamie, which is full of choking and darkness metaphors, despair and lack of hope and narrative wreckage, which means he lives with the *future in the present*, and with a present that is empty and static. The result is a fragmented self and the embodiment of chaos. Finally, the quest narrative contains journey metaphors, a sense of transcendent hope, and experiences of time in relation to fragmentary time, reclaimed time. And in this narrative the past is in the past, the present is in the present, and the future is in the future. Framed by this narrative and these notions of time, these kinds of metaphors, and this type of hope, SCI is reconfigured as a challenge and an opening to other ways of being as part of a developing self and a more communicative body.

Regardless of whether life is a narrative or narrative is a life, it would seem that narratives *do* matter for these men in the face of a disruptive and turning point moment in their lives. Indeed, they are an important productive practice for this group of men, after having become disabled through sport. Furthermore, the stories told here reveal that narratives are a useful, humane, even poetically inspired vehicle for conveying some of the richness, depth and profundity of the human experience to both the storyteller and the listener.[27] Notably, this dynamic process is embodied. Thus, not only do narratives matter, but the materiality of our individual fleshy bodies as biological entities and our bodies as socially constructed storied projects, also matter. This said, it should be acknowledged that the findings presented here are illuminative rather than definitive. Accordingly, the findings need to be treated with caution and seen as a point of departure for stimulating further questions and investigation. Questions remain, for example, regarding the processes by which the men in our study were drawn toward one particular narrative type over others and how shifts in each of these occur. Also, there needs to be a better understanding of how different types of self, metaphors, notions of time, and certain kinds of hope, congregate and coalesce within the restitution, chaos and quest narratives over time, and are performed in various contexts before different audiences. This is particularly so given the social nature of storytelling and the power differentials involved in this process, which allow some stories to be told and listened to while others are silenced or ignored. Clearly, it is beyond the scope of this chapter to address such issues. It remains, however, that narrative matters in the lives of individuals and needs to be taken seriously.

References

1 Frank AW (1995) *The Wounded Storyteller: body, illness and ethics.* The University of Chicago Press, Chicago.
2 Sparkes A (1998) Athletic identity: an Achilles heel to the survival of self. *Qual Health Res.* **8**: 644–64.

3 Seymour W (2002) Time and the body: re-embodying time in disability. *Journal of Occupational Science*. **9**: 135–42.

4 Medved M and Brockmeier J (2004) Making sense of traumatic experiences: telling a life with fragile X syndrome. *Qual Health Res*. **14**: 741–59.

5 Murray M (2003) Narrative psychology. In: J Smith (ed). *Qualitative Psychology*. Sage, London.

6 Brockmeier J and Carbaugh D (2001) Introduction. *Narrative and Identity: studies in autobiography, self and culture*. John Benjamins, Amsterdam/Philadelphia.

7 Miller P (1994) Narrative practices: their role in socialisation and self construction. In: U Neisser and R Fivush (eds). *The Remembering Self*. Cambridge University Press, Cambridge.

8 Murray M (1999) The storied nature of health and illness. In: M Murray and K Chamberlain (eds). *Qualitative Health Psychology*. Sage, London.

9 Somers M (1994) The narrative constitution of identity: a relational and network approach. *Theory Soc*. **23**: 635–49.

10 Connell R (1995) *Masculinities*. Polity Press, Cambridge.

11 Watson J (2000) *Male Bodies*. Open University Press, Buckingham.

12 Smith S and Watson J (2001) *Reading Autobiography*. University of Minnesota Press, Minneapolis.

13 Smith B and Sparkes A (2002) Men, sport, spinal cord injury, and the construction of coherence: narrative practice in action. *Qualitative Research*. **2**: 143–71.

14 Smith B and Sparkes A (2004) Men, sport, and spinal cord injury: an analysis of metaphors and narrative types. *Disabil Soc*. **19**: 509–612.

15 Smith B and Sparkes A. Men, sport, spinal cord injury and narratives of hope. *Social Science and Medicine* (in press).

16 Sparkes A (1999) Exploring body narratives. *Sport, Education and Society*. **4**: 17–30.

17 Sparkes A. Narrative analysis: exploring the *whats* and *hows* of personal stories. In: I Holloway (ed). *Qualitative Research in Health Care*. Open University Books, Buckingham (in press).

18 Sparkes A and Smith B (2002) Sport, spinal cord injuries, embodied masculinities, and narrative identity dilemmas. *Men and Masculinities*. **4**: 258–85.

19 Sparkes A and Smith B (2003) Men, sport, spinal cord injury and narrative time. *Qualitative Research*. **3**: 295–320.

20 Crossley M (2000) *Introducing Narrative Psychology*. Open University Press, Buckingham.

21 Roberts B (1999) Some thoughts on time perspectives and auto/biography. *Auto/Biography*. **VII**: 21–5.

22 Charmaz K (1991) *Good Days, Bad Days: the self in chronic illness and time*. Rutgers University Press, New Brunswick, NJ.

23 Marcel G (1962) *Homo Viator* [trans Craufurd E]. Harper and Row, New York.

24 Barnard D (1995) Chronic illness and the dynamics of hoping. In: K Toombs, D Barnard and R Carson (eds). *Chronic Illness: from experience to policy*. Indiana University Press, Bloomington.

25 Charmaz K (1987) Struggling for a self: identity levels of the chronically ill. In: J Roth and P Conrad (eds). *Research in the Sociology of Health Care: a research manual* [vol 6]. JAI Press Inc, Greenwich, CT.

26 Brockmeier J (2000) Autobiographical time. *Narrative Inquiry*. **19**: 51–73.

27 Freeman M (2003) When the story's over: narrative foreclosure and the possibility of self renewal. In: M Andrews, S Day Sclater and C Squire *et al* (eds). *Lines of Narrative*. Routledge, London.

Chapter 5

Body and self: a phenomenological study on the aging body and identity

Jennifer Bullington

Introduction

The process of aging cannot be understood merely in biological terms but must be seen as a complex social and psychological phenomenon where biology, psychology and culture all play a part in constituting the meaning of 'growing old'.[1] Accordingly, aging research does not focus exclusively on lack, disengagement and disability, topics that have been traditionally associated with old age. A modern research area is the investigation of the positive identity of the healthy, economically secure 'third age' retirement generation.[2–4] Aged individuals give meaning to their life situation in a variety of ways, and we see a variety of different cultures of aging.[3,5] Lifestyle analyses and research on consumerism is one way to understand the creation of identity in modern culture.[6,7] Anti-aging strategies and products show clearly how the desire to maintain control and ward off a negative self-image are important aspects of the creation of post-retirement identity.[8,9] Retired people in Western society today often have good enough health and economic resources to be able to pursue leisure activities which had not been possible for earlier generations. Taking care of one's body plays an important part in this self-creating project and many consumer activities are directed towards taking care of the body in order to achieve a sense of wellbeing, self-confidence and self-realisation.[10–12]

It has also been shown that older people's pessimistic beliefs about their health and ability to control the decline of the aging body contribute to the actual loss of function later on in life.[8] The role of activity and agency are important factors that are said to counter a negative downward spiral. To be able to organise one's life, have a variety of different experiences, regulate affect and motivate one's behaviour is necessary in order to be able to maintain a functional self.[13] Although there are some who see the emphasis placed upon activity for the elderly as a neo-liberal discourse that says more about our society than the needs of the aging,[14] the role of activity does seem to play an important part in contemporary research on aging. Thus, the importance of the body, either as the presented surface of self or the facilitator of activity, suggests that we should focus attention upon the aging body in order to deepen our understanding of the experience of 'growing old'. Self and body are intimately connected. But the 'body' which is of interest in this study is not the objective, naturalistic body – as understood and described within the natural sciences – but rather the 'lived body',[15–17] the embodied human being living in a meaningful context or life world. Much of the research on the body, in both medicine and sociology, has neglected the lived life world experience of the informants (for interesting exceptions, see Fleming,[18] Longino and Powell,[19] and Wainwright and Turner[20]). The body is either understood as a machine (as in traditional biomedicine) or as a field of play for socially constructed power discourses. The alternative that will enable us to catch the lived experience is phenomenology. Phenomenology is the systematic study of experience and subjectivity, an approach that will enable us to investigate the way in which the aging body is experienced. In this study, the role of the aging body in relation to identity and sense of self is explored.

The aim of the study

The aim of this study was to investigate how older people experience the aging body, and how these experiences affect aged people's sense of who they are. Special attention is paid to how bodily experiences are lived and described in relation to sense of self.

Method

Phenomenological method

The method of analysis used in this study was the Empirical Phenomenological Psychological method, the so-called EPP-method.[21] Phenomenological methods are based upon phenomenological philosophy. Phenomenology is a movement within continental philosophy that began with the works of the German philosopher Edmund Husserl[22] around the turn of the last century. The word 'phenomenology' means literally the logos of appearance. Phenomenology is concerned with the discovery of the essences, or the discovery of the meaning structure of phenomena. Phenomenological researchers do not attempt to validate hypothesis or prove theoretical constructions. In this tradition importance is placed upon openness to that which shows itself, to that which is 'given' in and through experience. All phenomenological methods, regardless of the technical procedure, are performed within the so-called 'phenomenological attitude' where the researcher 'brackets' or puts aside all presuppositions, theories and ideas about the phenomenon in question, in order to be open to the phenomenon as it appears. Obviously, a researcher approaches his or her subject of interest with a variety of ideas and questions concerning the phenomenon under study, but these interests are made consciously explicit so as to control for unwarranted bias in the interpretation of the data. Openness to the data and a descriptive, theory-neutral attitude characterises the phenomenological orientation. In this study, preconceived notions about aging and aging bodies were problematised so that that the informants could describe their experiences in a spontaneous non-directed way. The interview questions (Appendix A) were open-ended, in order to stimulate concrete detailed accounts of experience. The analysis technique in the EPP-method is composed of five analytic steps, designed to condense and draw out the themes and constituents that make up the meaning structure of the phenomenon in question. A hermeneutical moment is put into play when the empirical material is transformed into the researcher's perspective (from the informant's perspective) and when the meaning structure of the various interviews is constructed from the condensed situated structures (each interview analysed in light of the phenomenon in question). All interviews are collected before the analysis begins; however, it is possible to return to informants for a further interview in order to clarify or deepen themes or issues that have arisen from the analysis of the interviews. The findings from all interviews are presented in terms of either a general structure (if all interviews exhibit the same meaning structure) or in terms of typologies, where essential differences are maintained. See Karlsson[21] for detailed explication of the EPP-method.

Procedure

This study recruited informants from a retired people's organisation, two parishes in two different churches and a small number of informants still at work. The head of the retired people's organisation provided names and telephone numbers and e-mail to potential informants whom he imagined would be interested in participating in the study. Before making contact with these people, the researcher sent over written information about the study, which was posted at the main location of the retired people's meeting house. Some of these informants made contact with the researcher on the basis of the written information. The same procedure was followed in respect of the churches (the vicars providing the potential contacts). The small number of informants who were still at work were chosen by the researcher in terms of different means of employment. No one who was contacted declined the interview and none had misunderstood the aim of the study (to investigate experiences of aging with focus on the experience of the aging body). The informant categories were chosen in order to obtain data from people with different lifestyles and in different phases of the retirement/post-retirement life. Informants from the retired people's organisation were chosen in order to collect data about the experience of activity as an aged person, as one may imagine that people who join such an organisation have an interest in and capacity for activity despite old age. The church informants were chosen in order to catch spiritual, existential aspects of the aging experience. The reason that churchgoing informants were chosen to reflect these aspects was that it was assumed the issue of identity could be more easily explored in relation to spirituality if this dimension of life was organised socially through a parish affiliation. Those nearing retirement could shed light on the impending life change from work to retirement. The inclusion criteria for participation in the study were that the informant should be over 60 years of age and belong one of the three recruitment categories. Thirteen informants were interviewed (four men and nine women between the ages of 63 and 82, median age 69). The informants in this qualitative study were chosen in order to explore a diversity and richness in experience rather than providing a basis for statistical analysis or general conclusions about churchgoing people, men contra women, etc. Informants came from two cities in Sweden, one large city and one smaller town. The informants consisted of those persons who volunteered to be interviewed from the various recruitment categories. Their cultural background was Scandinavian. The open-ended, semi-structured interviews were tape-recorded and then transcribed for analysis. Each interview took approximately one hour. The interviews took place at the researcher's office, church location and in some instances at the workplace of the informant.

Results

No general structure was found which could take into account all the various meanings that imbued the 13 interviews. However, there was a general theme running through all the interviews concerning the experience of aging and the aged body which had to do with the experience of a changed life world, reactions to these changes in terms of body and self, and finding ways to feel at home in this changed life situation. This theme, found in all interviews, had to do with the experience that life was no longer as it had been, although the passage from 'before' to 'being old' differed from person to person. For some it was a powerful, shocking realisation, for others a gradual, almost imperceptible crossing over. The experience of the aging body was not always the most salient aspect of feeling like an old person, although all informants felt that their bodies were a reminder, in one way or another, that they were no longer young.

The results of this study will be presented below in terms of three typologies, reflecting the different ways in which these informants experienced the life world change brought about by aging, the reactions to this change in terms of body and self, and the way in which they found ways to feel at home in this new situation as an old person. The informants at times exhibited constituents from more than one typology, although each informant had a basic style to their experience corresponding to one of the three typologies. The typologies presented in detail below have been called 'Existential awakening', 'Making it good enough' and 'New possibilities'. The quotations from the interviews are cited in terms of interview number followed by page number in the interview, e.g. [I9:12].

Typology I: 'Existential awakening' (2 female informants)

The change (typology I)

The experience of aging was both shocking and completely unexpected. An element of surprise and horror was experienced in connection with becoming an old person. That which had been previously taken for granted (such as taking responsibility as a boss, being attractive to the opposite sex) was now gone. The experience of loss was profound since the informants realised that they had not appreciated what they had until it was gone.

> It's sad in that I hadn't understood, when I was young and I suppose I was pretty then, I had quite a few suitors. I have always had a lot of men around me and I was married many years, but I wasn't happy about that then. But today it's all gone, and I see that it's gone and I see that I had it then... *[I13: 3]*

There was an awareness of death approaching on the horizon and these informants were directed towards this coming event, although neither was in ill health. They were grappling with the realisation that life was approaching its final phase. This process was described by one of the same informants as above in the following way:

> I am freeing myself slowly from everything that has tied me to life. I have danced, had a good time, been married, loved my beautiful home, but I think now, you can just put everything you have in two plastic bags and just go. *[I13: 3]*

Things that had seemed important before were now found to be inessential. There was a directing of attention towards 'things that mattered', such as close relationships. Questions having to do with the finitude of life and death were actualised, which gave a sense of resoluteness to this phase of life. Insights about oneself were accepted, even if they were painful:

> Before I had always believed that I had really bad self-confidence, but I can see now that I was very competent. I had never believed that I was intellectual or good at reading, but now I have discovered, I have been able to get a whole bunch of stipendiums. *[17: 14–15]*

The physical dimension of aging was not as pronounced as the existential aspects of becoming old.

Reactions in terms of body and self (typology I)

These informants did not like their aging bodies, found them unattractive and not corresponding to their feelings of being themselves. The decline of their faculties (memory, physical ability) was experienced as 'terrible'. However, the aging body was experienced as a surface seen by others, not as the self. Descriptions of the body's unattractiveness in the interviews were immediately followed by descriptions of self-affirmation, in contrast to the unattractive appearance, as can be seen in the following excerpts:

> Today I have great trouble getting myself to put on a bathing suit. I see that my legs have tremendous varicose veins and I look just awful you know…but I love the clear water and sun, because I love nature and I lie there with the wind and sun, so close to my Lord and I think when I lie there that there is some kind of inebriated moment that is healing, you know, even if I am ugly and skinny and yuck old and haven't got any money and everything has just gone to hell, but lying there I am so infinitely happy in all the beauty, the beauty. *[I13: 8]*

> I don't like the way I look nowadays. I don't like my body, that's the long and short of it. I swim and ride my bike, I get up at 5.30 every morning, ride my bike to the lake and swim every morning out there where I live. And I have a summer cottage in *[X]* where I spend the summers, and there I am the only one in the whole village who takes a dip, even in the winter. *[I7: 5]*

Feeling at home as old (typology I)

The way of coping with the unattractive, aged body and the existential issues presented above could be described in this typology as moving towards transcendence, or more plainly, moving out of oneself. Because the body (as surface) is no longer a source of positive self-image, there is a tendency to not pay so much attention to the body or even to the self. There is a movement away from self towards others. For one informant, this other is God, in the other informant's interview she describes how she has filled her time after retirement with a variety of volunteer activities. The transcendence movement was not conscious coping strategy, but rather arose as a consequence of the existential awakening. The resoluteness felt in relation to the realisation of the finitude of life led to an insight that the important things should be prioritised, important things having to do with non-material aspects of life such as close relationships, God, taking care of others in need. One is 'at home' in being for the other. This style or way of being for the other will be contrasted to a similar constituent in typology III (*New possibilities*), where the motivation and driving force is of a different character.

Typology II: 'Making it good enough' (three female informants)

The change (typology II)

The informants in this category experienced most profoundly the changes in their bodies due to the aging process. While the informants in the previous typology did not speak so often about their bodies during the interview (besides the few comments about how they found their bodies basically unattractive), these three informants dealt extensively with how the aging body gave rise to new experiences, both good and bad. One informant had discovered that she no longer felt that she had to worry about prestige and could experience that being an older person gave her permission to be a bit childish. Because she could no longer 'keep up' with the pace of younger people, due to her aging body and its failure, she felt a new freedom in relation to achievements. A feeling of wonder could come over her from time to time, as she saw things in a new way, almost as a child. She related how she and her husband were on a walk one day when they saw two big birds circling overhead:

> They swayed up and down and came very close to us, we were standing still, so maybe they thought we were prey, but they had these big white and black wings, so fantastic to see such birds here, that we had never seen before. It was fun, sort of childish, and we said 'it doesn't matter that we stand here like this because we're old people, nobody cares about us if we stand here like this and just look'. *[I9: 6]*

A negative experience related to the aging body was the fear of travelling. One informant had travelled extensively in her youth, but was now afraid to travel because she didn't want to become ill or in need of help being far away from home. This same person remarked that it was much harder for her now to learn new things. She noticed how her granddaughter had a much easier time learning Spanish when they took a Spanish class together. She needed to write things down in order to not forget. She had become a bit lazy and had a harder time to motivate herself to do things, since she didn't *have* to do anything anymore.

Reactions in terms of body and self (typology II)

The aging body was experienced as an antagonist for these informants. Their bodies disobeyed them in various ways, the hands that 'won't do what I want anymore' [I9: 1], the 'body on strike' [I11: 1]. The body could be experienced as alien, 'My body is not me' [I9: 7], 'My body doesn't do what I want to do' [I9: 3]. The emphasis here was not on the changed appearance of the body (as in typology I) but rather on the diminished strength and control the informants experienced in relation to their bodies. They were keenly aware that the weakness of the body prevented them from doing what they would like to do. There was a battle going on between self and body, where the self had no choice but to capitulate. One could no longer do exercise as before, one had to take into consideration back pain, worn out joints, etc. Aches and pains of the body were discussed in relation to concrete activities that the informants would like to do, but were not able to do anymore because of the body.

> One warm summer my little grandson spurted me with a water pistol and I ran, it was warm out and he ran after me, it was such fun. Then a few years later he said, 'Grandma, let's run again!' and I said, 'No, you know Grandma can't run anymore, I am getting a bit old' and he said, 'Grandma, you remember how you ran,' he remembered that, I said, 'Yes, but I'm not going to do that now.' *[I9: 3]*

At times one informant related how she could decide to defy the limitations of her aging body, but afterwards had to pay a price:

> I still take walks *[despite arthritis in the knees]*, if I decide I want to do something, I just do it, but then I have to pay for it with pain afterwards, but most often it's worth it. *[I11: 1]*

Feeling at home as old (typology II)

The theme running through these interviews could be called 'making it good enough'. The failing body interferes with the will and desires of the self, which calls for some kind of coping strategy. These informants expressed that they tried to make the best of the situation, trying to find things to be grateful for every day, or just being thankful for the time one has left to live, one day at a time. One informant found a new goal in life, starting up a new activity programme for youth in her town, which she did in her own way, at her own pace. It was a bit of a challenge to take on this responsibility, and she had to weigh the pros and cons in relation to her physical and mental capacity as an older, retired person:

> I though, oh boy, that would be great fun to be a part of, but I can't keep up with it, no, that wouldn't be possible because you have classes all day on Mondays and half of Tuesday and other days, but they had taken into account that I felt very strongly for this kind of activity, they said, of course you can do this, and now I am sitting there with 6–7 young people! It is very, very fun, really, but it is tiring. *[I9: 2]*

> One has to lower the level of ambition and try to make do with what is possible, I have become so tired that I can't take exercise class any more, I have pain in my back, it is hard and that's probably why I've gotten so stiff in my body too. When I went into retirement, I worked until I was 65, I started to go to this Senior exercise class, done that a few years, water aerobics too, but I can't do that anymore, because I've gotten so stiff in my body, but now I try to just move around as much as I can, go and take walks and so on. *[I6: 1]*

This phase of life involved limitations for them, but they did not experience sadness or anxiety about the coming nearer to the end of life. Neither did they express the existential concerns which characterised the informants in typology I.

Typology III: 'New possibilities' (4 female and 4 male informants)

The change (typology III)

All of the male informants belong to this typology. The most striking aspect of change that came through in these interviews had to do with the joy experienced in relation to new possibilities that aging (being retired or semi-retired) opened up. The informants often referred to how wonderful it was to be free, to not have to conform to the rules and regulations of working life. One gets up when one wishes, does what one wants during the day, one decides when one wants to go home, when one goes out and so on. Being retired was a 'luxury' [I12: 10]. The passage from working life to retirement was not the great overwhelming divide that some had expected, rather a surprisingly easy passage. None of the informants missed their jobs, although they all spoke of how they had enjoyed their work. The most appreciated aspect of being retired was being free. The informants spoke primarily about changes in attitude (life philosophy) and in some cases changes in personality rather than bodily changes, although there were aches and pains and somatic difficulties. Several (female) informants related how they had learned to say no to others, and to not care so much about what others think:

> It's almost a bit comic, I think, that when you get older you don't have to be as careful as before. I find that to be a liberating feeling. I must say that I dare more to say what I think today. *[I4: 5]*

> One doesn't feel the same kind of pressure from people in a way, like before I thought that you had to achieve and all that, now I just do what I feel like, and I don't care so much what other people think. *[I5: 5]*

Aging had brought about a sense of calmness, where one felt less restless and dissatisfied. In general, it would seem that the experience of aging for this group gave rise to an acceptance of the way things are, on all levels (physical, mental, social). The way in which these informants spoke about 'acceptance' differed from the acceptance found in typology II. That which was characteristic for the way in which these informants spoke about acceptance was that acceptance here did not have the same coping function that it had in typology II (*Making it good enough*), where acceptance was a strategy used to deal with an antagonist body. Here acceptance seemed to be rather a philosophy of life:

> I have the insight that I am getting old, and I accept that. I know that I will have less and less energy and all that, but I see it as a part of a natural process. *[I3: 4]*

Informants were oriented towards the future, although not towards the approaching of death. The future was imagined as filled with pleasant activities.

Reactions in terms of body and self (typology III)

The bodily changes discussed in these interviews had to do with the same kinds of experiences brought up in the previous typologies, such as gaining weight, getting wrinkles, feeling less attractive, loss of energy, aches and pains, failing mental faculties. However, the attitude to these bodily changes was marked by acceptance, as described above. The body showed definite signs of aging, but the response to these changes was to not pay too much attention to the body:

> I don't think about *[my appearance]* so much, I usually say, I am the way I am, we all have to get old. Wrinkles aren't that bad, everybody get them, and there's nothing you can do about it. *[I1: 10]*

> There are always some extra pounds, one lives a good life. I try now and then to hold back on the food, but it's nothing that I suffer from or anything like that. *[I5: 3]*

The aging body did not influence the way these informants felt about themselves, they were at home in their bodies in a way that the informants in the previous typologies were not. The body was still a source of pleasure (eating and drinking, relaxing, taking vacations, etc.) despite signs of aging. Where the informants in typology II did battle with their bodies, these informants were at peace with their bodies, as they did not experience their bodies as something alien from themselves.

Feeling at home as old (typology III)

The common thread running through these interviews had to do with the importance of activity for wellbeing. As one (male) informant expressed it:

> Well, you have to get some interests and realise yourself in a new way, you can't feel proud of yourself about working life any more, now you have to feel proud about the fact that you can help out with volunteer work, do something in the Church, and help your children and grandchildren when they need it, that gives me an identity today. *[I10: 3]*

Being active was seen as a way to not give in to depressing thoughts and self-preoccupation. One informant stated that he must have a daily programme, for otherwise he would become ill. Being active was a way for informants to ward off a negative spiral, resulting in isolation and illness. It was not good enough to just sit at home or restrict oneself to the company of one's own family. One should have something to look forward to during the week, like meeting a friend, going to a concert, helping out at church, etc. Being-for-others was one way to keep in shape (cf. self-transcendence in typology I). The theme of positive thinking was pronounced in this group of informants. One had a responsibility to take advantage of all that life has to offer. The informants enjoyed ordinary everyday things, like drinking wine at dinner on a weekday. They reported that they lived a very pleasant life. The informants in this category were reflective to varying degrees, some had never thought of illness or death, others were aware that aging brings one closer to the end of life. But none were grappling with the existential issues that the informants in typology I were dealing with. The focus in this group was upon the advantages of retirement (and semi-retirement) as freedom and possibility, rather than dwelling on the limitations of the body or existential issues. They said that they felt as if they had been given a long vacation to enjoy, which they did to a high degree.

Discussion

We see in the above typologies three different possible ways of experiencing the aged body and self. The relevant aspects or themes that emerged from the analysis have to do with the general theme found regarding the experiences of life world change, reactions to change in terms of body and self and ways of feeling at home in the changed life situation that aging brings about. In the first typology *Existential awakening*, we see the most dramatic experience of this change, with a profound reorientation in terms of priorities. The existential themes of loss, remorse and resoluteness were pronounced in these interviews. The body was rarely mentioned, but when it came up in the interview it had to do with how unattractive the body had become. The body and self were transcended for these informants in a way of feeling at home that involved focusing on the other.

In the typology *Making it good enough*, the most salient recurring constituent had to do with battling the aging body, the body which is no longer 'me'. These informants did not have more severe health problems than informants in the other typologies, but they experienced frustration in relation to the limitations imposed by the aging body in a way that was especially pronounced in this group. They were not concerned with physical appearance (cf. *Existential awakening*) so much as their reduced physical and mental capabilities. The limitations of the body stood in the way of the will, which gave rise to the need for a coping strategy. These informants decided to 'make the best of it' and could even find some advantages to being an elderly person. On one level they seemed to accept the changes and limitations brought about by aging, but yet they still 'did battle' with the body in a way in which the others did not.

The third typology, *New possibilities*, provides the strongest contrast to the previous typologies. Here we see neither existential issues nor battles with the body. These informants felt at one with their bodies, enjoyed the freedom they experience as retired (or semi-retired) and seemed at peace with being an old person. They had fully accepted the aging process and their aging bodies. However, several informants in this typology stressed the importance of positive thinking, which suggests that the peace and acceptance was something they had to work at. They were aware that they used activities as a way to stay in shape and prevent feelings of isolation and depression. All the men in this study belonged to this typology. Although these informants were by no means oblivious to the fact that aging brought them closer to the end of life, they had no special feelings or thoughts about this.

What do these three typologies tell us about the way in which the aging body impacts on experiences of self and the life world? Using the results as descriptions of *possible ways* in which the phenomenon of the aging body in relation to identity appears, we can see that the mere fact of having aches and pains and age-related limitations did not automatically result in negative experiences of self. We have also seen that the informants in this study had different ways of constituting the meaning of their aging bodies. Only in one typology (*Making it good enough*) did the informants express marked frustration over their limitations and felt the need to develop coping strategies. Likewise, it was only in one typology (*Existential awakening*) that we saw that changed physical appearance (experienced as unattractive) played a role in self-perception. Wrinkles and extra kilos were of no special importance to the informants in *New possibilities*. The importance of activity for wellbeing was seen most clearly in the typology *New possibilities*, where an emphasis was placed upon freedom, responsibility and positive thinking. Activity for these informants was one of several ways to take charge of one's life and keep in shape. The motivation for the activity engaged in by the informants in the other two typologies came from either the existential insight that life is short and coming to an end (*Existential awakening*) or the philosophical attitude that you have to make the best of what you have, from day to day, adjusting your activity to your capabilities (*Making it good enough*).

None of the informants spoke about consumer activities or products in their interviews. One female informant said that she thought it was important to have nice clothes, and a male informant remarked that he had found that he was treated better (as an older person) if he had on a suit and tie, but all in all the informants did not use products or consumption in order to create or strengthen a sense of self. Feeling at home as an old person for these informants had to do with finding self-esteem in relationships (specifically in close relationships with relatives and friends, or with God) or in various types of volunteer activities or leisure activities. The leisure activities which came up in the interviews were, for example, drinking coffee with friends, going dancing, taking walks, playing golf, going to the country cottage, swimming and taking vacations. Some of these activities required having money, while others did not. The informants in the typology *New possibilities* spoke the most about leisure activities, and the informants in *Existential awakening* the least.

Concluding remarks

The results from this study could be said to give support to the research that points out the importance of activity for the self-esteem of the elderly. All informants spoke of activity in relation to post- or near post-retirement identity, either the projects motivated by anticipatory resoluteness in *Existential awakening*, the importance of day-to-day activity in *Making it good enough*, or the importance of leisure activity/charity activity for wellbeing in *New Possibilities*. However, we have seen that 'activity' can mean different things to different people and have different sources of motivation. The influence of the aging body on sense of self and identity was illustrated by three different typologies, where only one group expressed frustration over the limitations of the aging body. Only this group of informants experienced the body as 'not-me'. Why this was so would be interesting to penetrate further. What does it mean to experience alienation from one's body as an older person? What are the factors that allow people to maintain a positive sense of self and identity despite failing faculties and changed physical appearance? Another interesting finding was that informants in two typologies exhibited entirely different ways of relating to the fact that death is approaching (*Existential awakening* and *New possibilities*), which raises questions about how older people experience this impending horizon.

Finally, the gender differences between men and women in this small study were quite clear, where all the male informants belonged to the typology *New possibilities*. A further investigation of how males and females experience different aspects of the aging process could be a topic for future phenomenological studies, with emphasis placed upon the meaning of freedom, appearance, activity and self-esteem.

Acknowledgements

I would like to thank the research group at the Institute for the Study of Ageing and Later Life (ISAL) at the Department of Thematic Studies, Linköping University, Campus Norrköping, for their support during the initial phase of this study. I would also like to thank Professor Gunnar Karlsson for valuable comments on the manuscript and a special thanks to all the informants who spoke with me freely and inspiringly about their experiences of aging and identity.

References

1 Williams S and Bendelow G (1998) *The Lived Body: sociological themes, embodied issues.* Routledge, London.
2 Gilleard C and Higgs P (2000) *Cultures of Aging: self, citizen and the body.* Prentice Hall, Harlow.
3 Hendricks J and Cutler SJ (1990) Leisure and the structure of our life worlds. *Aging and Society.* **10**: 85–94.
4 Laslett P (1989) *A Fresh Map of Life: the emergence of the third age.* Weidenfeld & Nicolson, London.
5 Thompson P (1993) 'I don't feel old': the significance of the search for meaning in later life. *International Journal of Geriatric Psychiatry.* **8**: 685–92.
6 Giddens A (1991) *Modernity and Self-Identity: self and society in the late modern age.* Polity Press, Cambridge.
7 Öberg P and Tornstam L (1999) Body images among men and women at different ages. *Aging and Society.* **19**: 629–44.
8 Boult C, Altman M, Gilbertson D *et al* (1996) Decreasing disability in the 21st century. *American Journal of Public Health.* **86**: 1388–93.
9 Levy B and Langer E (1994) Aging free from negative stereotypes: successful memory in China and among the American deaf. *Journal of Personality and Social Psychology.* **66**: 989–97.
10 Featherstone M and Hepworth M (1991) The mask of aging and the post-modern life course. In: M Featherstone, M Hepworth and BS Turner (eds). *The Body: social process and cultural theory.* Sage, London.
11 Hennessy CA (1989) Culture in the use, care and control of the aging body. *Journal of Aging Studies.* **3**(1): 39–54.
12 Shilling C (1993) *The Body and Social Theory.* Sage, London.
13 Markus HR and Herson AR (1992) The role of the self-concept in aging. *Annual Review of Gerontology and Geriatrics.* **11**: 110–43.
14 Katz S (2000) Busy bodies: activity, aging and the management of everyday life. *Journal of Aging Studies.* **14**(2): 135–52.
15 Bullington J (1999) *The Mysterious Life of the Body: a new look at psychosomatics.* Almqvist & Wiksell International, Stockholm.
16 Merleau-Ponty M (1942/1963) *The Structure of Behavior.* Beacon Press, Boston.
17 Merleau-Ponty M (1945/1962) *Phenomenology of Perception.* Routledge & Kegan Paul, London.

18 Fleming AA (2001) Older men 'working it out: ' a strong face of aging and disability. Doctoral dissertation, University of Sydney, Australia, School of Behavioral and Community Health Services.

19 Longino CF and Powell JL (2003) Embodiment and the study of aging. In: V Berdayes (ed). *The Body in Human Inquiry: interdisciplinary explorations of embodiment.* Research publication at Salford Centre for Gerontological studies (SCGS), University of Salford.

20 Wainwright SP and Turner BS (2003) Reflections on embodiment and vulnerability. *J Med Ethics; Medical Humanities*: 4–7.

21 Karlsson G (1995) *Psychological Qualitative Research from a Phenomenological Perspective.* Almqvist & Wiksell International, Göteborg.

22 Husserl E (1913/1962) *Ideas: general introduction to pure phenomenology, Vol 1.* Collier Books, New York.

Appendix A

Interview guide (translated from Swedish)

General instruction: Tell me about concrete experiences you come to think of in relation to the interview questions, and relate these experiences in as much detail as possible. What happened? What did you think? How did you feel? What was going on? and so forth. There is no right or wrong answer, so anything you want to tell me about is quite all right.

Introductory question

First of all I would like to ask you a little bit about what it's like for you to age? How do you experience your own aging? Was it how you thought it would be? Tell me about it.

Body

1 Can you tell me about a concrete situation when you first understood that your body was aging? How could you tell, what did you think/feel at that time?

2 Do you feel at peace with your body? Do you feel that your body prevents you from doing things, or influences you in one way or another in your daily life?

3 Do you feel your age? How old do you feel?

Identity

1 Can you describe for me a situation where you felt that you really gave expression to who you are, that is to say, in this situation you felt as if your personality and self came through? [Do they take an experience from the past, recent past? If long ago, ask if there are situations closer to the present, and compare theses two examples.] Alternative question: Is there something that is typically *you*, can you describe a situation for me when this characteristic became very prominent?

2 Can you give me an example of a situation where you felt that you were not really yourself, where you felt false or untrue to yourself [as above]?

Body and identity

1 Have you changed you opinion of yourself, who you are, since you have become older? If this is the case, does your body or your appearance have anything to do with this?

2 Can you tell me about how you see yourself now, in this current life phase, in relation to how you saw yourself as a younger person? Can you exemplify? [Notice the body in these examples.]

Finally, I wonder if there is something you would like to add that you can think of now that we have not talked about in this interview?

Thank you so much for your participation!

Chapter 6

Self and narrative in schizophrenia: time to author a new story

David Roe and Larry Davidson

There are a couple of reasons why the topic for this chapter may strike some readers as curious. Given the focus of this book, it will not be the interest in narrative or self which will be unexpected, of course, but the notion that these concepts could have relevance within the context of a disease as disruptive and devastating as schizophrenia. While other people can write narratives *about* persons who have schizophrenia – like Nassar's[1] recent biography of Nobel laureate John Nash – the idea that a person with schizophrenia would construct his own narrative may seem at first counterintuitive. Since it was first identified as the most severe of the mental illnesses over a century ago, schizophrenia has been described not only as a loss of sanity but also as a loss of one's sense of self at the most fundamental level of self-awareness.[2,3] The third edition of the *Diagnostic and Statistical Manual of Mental Disorders* of the American Psychiatric Association, for example, suggests that 'the sense of self that gives the normal person a feeling of individuality, uniqueness, and self direction is frequently disturbed in schizophrenia'.[4] If people with schizophrenia lose this kind of sense of themselves as people, as agents of their own lives, how could they possibly author their own stories?

In addition to the concern about loss of self, the clinical literature on schizophrenia has suggested that one of the core elements of the thought disorder associated with this condition is the diminished capacity of people with schizophrenia to create coherent narratives about their lives.[5] While some earlier representatives of the antipsychiatry movement suggested that this difficulty reflected fragmentation and incoherence in the person's familial environment rather than in the person,[3] other more recent theoreticians – reflecting a postmodernist consciousness – have suggested that this deficit is actually more of a (potential) asset.[6] In any case, regardless of the cause, even if people with schizophrenia do not entirely lose their sense of self, they would still seem to have lost the ability to compose temporally unified and coherent autobiographical accounts.[5] How, then, can they even construct, not to mention use to their benefit, narratives about their illness, their impact on sense of self, and their efforts to recover?

In the following, we intend to argue that these concerns about people with schizophrenia are only relevant – to the degree that they are relevant at all – to the more acute phases and/or severe forms of the disorder. In addition, we suggest that the emerging 'recovery' paradigm in community mental health opens an exciting new window onto the rich but relatively unexplored terrain of self and life reconstruction that occurs throughout the recovery process. Despite its bleak history as a progressive, deteriorating disease, we now know that over half of those individuals meeting diagnostic criteria for schizophrenia will demonstrate significant improvement over time, many recovering fully.[7] As a result of this research, we suggest that it is time to author a new story about schizophrenia; one in which recovery plays at least as prominent a role as disorder. Drawing on our own empirical research in this growing area, we describe the person's efforts to deal with the disruptions and discontinuities introduced by the illness, as well as her efforts to regain a sense of agency and a coherent life narrative in their wake. We suggest in closing that, rather than simply being a by-product of recovery, reconstructing a sense of social agency and re-authoring one's life story should be considered key dimensions of recovery which interact with other important domains in meaningful ways.

Schizophrenia and the negation of narrative

On what basis has the possibility of narrative been negated in the lives of people with schizophrenia? Schizophrenia is the medical term given by the field of psychiatry that most closely captures phenomena that otherwise would be described by the lay public as insanity or madness. Talking out loud to oneself (actually in response to hallucinated voices); holding firm to false and idiosyncratic – if not outright bizarre – notions; failing to attend to personal hygiene; mumbling incoherently; and being terrified by thoughts that others are trying to do one harm are among the characteristic features of this potentially devastating disease which affects one out of every 100 people. While historically there has never been a consensus on what causes this condition or where it comes from (competing explanations range from demonic possession and witchcraft to faulty parenting and biological deficits), there have been concrete effects for people who appear to have it. These have included stoning; burning at the stake; confinement in distant institutions; abandonment to the streets; and a variety of treatments such as electroconvulsive therapy and lobotomy. What all of these effects had in common was that they were based on the underlying belief that the person with schizophrenia lacks reason to such an extent that he is not even aware of his lack of reason. It has been on the basis of the perception that people with schizophrenia become totally absorbed into their illness and thus lose touch with reality, that both narrative and self have been negated, leaving behind nothing more than an 'empty shell' of a person.[8] Not only has this perception been shown to be false,[9] it also has the effect of further abandoning the person to the illness, dismissing rather than inviting narrative.

Even if the person remains behind or beneath the illness, the reader may object, surely he or she is unaware of the illness and its effects on her life. While she may still be able to tell stories, of what value could these stories be when they emanate from within the disorder? One important way in which attitudes toward schizophrenia have differed historically from other chronic illnesses has been the belief that people with schizophrenia are not aware of the fact that they have this condition and may even lack insight into the fact that they have any difficulties at all.[10] Were this true, it certainly would then be a challenge for people with schizophrenia to describe how the illness has affected their lives and sense of self, since they would be unaware of any such changes. Prior to disputing these claims, it will be useful for us to consider their source in the application, and limitations, of objective/descriptive psychiatry.

Objective/descriptive psychiatry, since publication of the third edition of the *Diagnostic and Statistical Manual of Mental Disorders*,[4] has attempted to eschew theory and a focus on the life experiences of people with mental illness in order to classify disorders based on what can be readily observed and measured. While establishing standardised measures and operational criteria for disorders has contributed to increasing the reliability of diagnostic concepts and improving communication among researchers, limiting psychiatric knowledge to what can be objectively described and measured has also made it difficult, if not impossible, for the field to consider a range of other potentially important data. Frank and Frank[11] point out, for example, that descriptive psychiatry's 'atheoretical' stance actually posits a theory in itself: that the meaning people attach to their symptoms, their beliefs about and attitudes toward their illness, and their social and historical context, are all unimportant. Carrying this argument a step further, Kleinman[12] emphasises the importance of engaging in participant observation to facilitate eliciting patients' explanatory models of illness in order to understand their own personal experiences and the social sources and consequences of those personal experiences.

Kleinman's argument, along with the more recent body of work on illness narratives,[13] models,[14,15] perceptions[16] and beliefs,[17] suggests that we may have overlooked an extremely important dimension of schizophrenia, which is to be found precisely in the person's experiences of the illness and its impact on his life. In suggesting that lack of awareness of illness, or 'anosognosia', is a core feature of schizophrenia, objective/descriptive psychiatrists overlooked the fact that it has only been very recently that we have begun to share our growing knowledge about the illness with the people who are seeking treatment. All during the previous 150 years of confinement and community care – the period during which the presumed lack of awareness of illness became established as a core feature of schizophrenia – it seldom occurred to practitioners to tell people with schizophrenia their diagnosis or to offer them information about the nature of mental illness and its treatment. Some of those few to whom it did occur were prohibited from doing so by virtue of their (psychodynamic) training, while others who offered people this information apparently did so in secret, so that we have no way of knowing the effect of such interventions on the person's degree of insight.[18] More recently, however, we have begun to provide information and education about schizophrenia and its treatment not only to people newly diagnosed with the condition, but even to people considered at risk of mental illness, and with good results.[19] What these findings suggest in retrospect is that we never should have expected people to be aware of the fact that they had a mental illness when we never offered them that information in the first place. This would be similar to speculating that lack of insight is intrinsic to cancer since people do not walk into their physician's office and report that they suspect they might be growing a tumour. Without any advance education, and in the face of hundreds of years of stigma, people experiencing mental illness had little reason to guess that what was afflicting them was a psychiatric disorder.

Does this mean that everyone who now develops schizophrenia will be educated about it, accept the diagnostic label, and demonstrate adequate insight into their need for treatment? No. What it does suggest, however, is that the difficulties they may encounter in accepting this diagnosis and adhering to a prescribed treatment regimen will be more alike than different from the difficulties encountered by people with other chronic illnesses. What may be more different in the case of schizophrenia is not so much the person as our own standards for acceptance or distortion of reality. That is, we seem to have a double standard pertaining to the wide range of socially acceptable ways we have to avoid the reality of our fundamental vulnerability, fragility and mortality. In the case of other chronic or terminal illnesses, we might refer to denial or lack of acceptance of our diagnosis or prognosis as a positive illusion.[20] We may be willing to lie, deceive or go out of our way to be elusive when interacting with a dying person. But in the case of mental illness, we insist that people accept their diagnostic label – with the good intention of improving adherence and outcome – and view their 'lack of insight' as further evidence of their condition. Such a position fails to appreciate the adaptive role played by denial in much of human experience, including in adaptation to illness.

Several recent studies have confirmed the negative relationship that may exist between the acceptance of a diagnostic label and aspects of psychosocial wellbeing and quality of life, particularly when self efficacy is low – as it often is in schizophrenia.[21–23] These studies suggest that one reason people with this condition may not wish to accept or discuss their diagnosis is that to do so leaves them feeling hopeless, helpless, and demoralised. In addition, there continues to be the issue of stigma. Even if I become educated about schizophrenia and accept that I have this condition, I remain aware of the fact that most people associate it with axe murderers, serial killers, or, at best, 'the mentally ill'. Being aware of my condition does not therefore necessarily translate into being willing to disclose that information to others.[24]

This should not come as a surprise, considering that disclosure often leads to the painful confrontation with society's prevailing stigma,[25,26] discrimination[27] and ignorance about mental illness. The devastating stigma is often further reinforced by the media[28] presenting stereotypical, usually negative, images of people with mental illness, turning them into 'the lepers of the twentieth century'.[29] No wonder 'having insight' or 'accepting' having a mental disorder is typically not an easy or linear process.

Where does this leave us? According to the objective/descriptive psychiatric model of schizophrenia, lack of insight is produced by an inability of the impaired brain to process data about its own dysfunction.[30] Once we accept this assumption, people are doomed to confirm their diagnosis regardless of how they react to the information they are given. If they accept the diagnosis, for instance, this constitutes their agreement, despite the fact that if they really do have the illness they are not supposed to be capable of having such awareness. Agreement also renders all of their other beliefs, ideas and decisions suspect at best, as we still view schizophrenia as impairing their cognitive abilities and judgment. If, on the other hand, they deny the diagnosis, or refuse to accept it, this act can be used as evidence that the person lacks insight and therefore must have a mental illness.[31] As a result, all of her beliefs, ideas and decisions are similarly suspect, if not dismissed out of hand. Either way, the person is viewed as lacking the essential prerequisites for being a narrator of her own experience: awareness and insight. Should the person nonetheless presume to offer an alternative narrative to the biomedical one, common responses to such narratives have been, according to Estroff, to 'frame them as denial, lack of insight, transference, or evidence in direct contradiction to the narrator's claim of validity'.[32] In the end, either way, narrative has been negated.

This position reflects the fact that objective/descriptive psychiatry has tended to equate insight with the person's ability to articulate the perspective of the clinician, even when this has not been shared with him or her directly,[33] resulting in an overly narrow view of awareness. In an earlier review,[34] we found, for example, that patients' and staff members' attitudes toward a wide range of treatment issues almost always diverged, irrespective of the topic, place, time, and demographic or clinical characteristics of the sample. In another study[35] we compared the perspectives of people hospitalised in a psychiatric facility with those of facility staff regarding the rights of hospitalised psychiatric patients. We found prevailing disagreement when treatment compromised patients' rights, with staff consistently preferring the treatment and patients preferring their rights.[35]

The importance of these findings is that they demonstrate that the perceptions of a person with a mental illness may or may not be a result of his disorder, or of the degree to which he has or lacks insight, but rather may simply reflect his own personal preferences. As such, these perceptions need not be challenged or changed until they match a correct or valid perception (which could be assumed to be that of the staff) but rather may represent a personal choice of equal validity. This shift from holding up a dominant worldview to which we expect all perspectives to correspond, to acknowledging the coexistence of multiple, diverse views may be a necessary precondition for encouraging people with schizophrenia to compose and share their narratives, and for these narratives to be respected, not only as valid and useful tools for research, but as a foundation for recovery as well.

Narratives of self and illness

So when offered the opportunity to compose and share their narratives, what do people with schizophrenia tell us?

Ridgway[36] analysed published first person accounts of recovery and emphasised broad common passages, including moving from despair to hope, from withdrawal to engagement, and from passive adjustment to active coping and the reclaiming of a positive sense of self, meaning, and purpose. In another study, Jacobson[37] analysed narratives of recovery using a dimensional analysis and identified component processes which corresponded to four central dimensions: recognising the problem; transforming the self; reconciling with the system; and reaching out to others.

Indeed, much of existing research on this topic suggests that people struggle with accepting and incorporating their illness as only one dimension of an expanded sense of self.[38] These discussions of the impact of psychiatric illness on the person's former sense of self already assume, however, that the person has been made aware of the fact that other people, particularly mental health professionals and family members, view what has been happening to them as indicative of their having a major mental illness. One of the first things people with schizophrenia tell us, however, when we ask them for stories about their illness and recovery is that they were not aware initially that what they were experiencing was in fact a mental illness. In fact, people with schizophrenia typically experience symptoms for months to years with the active illness before seeking or receiving treatment.[19] As we noted above, in the absence of education or other advance preparation, most people have no basis upon which to attribute their experiences of hearing voices, having strange but persistent ideas or having various cognitive difficulties to the onset of a mental illness. Little is known about what alternative explanations people develop in the absence of this kind of bio-medical knowledge.

What we are suggesting is that people with schizophrenia still need to find a way to make sense of these anomalous experiences even when they are left to their own devices. Contrary to the objective/descriptive approach described above, our experience suggests that people are indeed acutely aware of their increasing difficulties; it is just that they do not know how to account for them. What we have found thus far is that people eventually come up with highly individual – if not idiosyncratic – explanations based on their own prior experiences, religious and cultural affiliations, and social environments. Despite the uniquely personal nature of these explanations, several common themes have emerged. These include punishment for previous sins or transgression, as well as:

> religious accounts of such things as demonic possession or visitations by God; persecutory ideas about the activities of foreign powers, aliens, or various versions of the secret police (e.g., CIA or FBI agents); or more up to date beliefs about being under the influence of different forms of technology, such as computer chips implanted in the brain, infrared or ultraviolet surveillance, or electronic thought broadcasting.[24]

Within a clinical context, these types of explanations are often viewed as delusional ideas that are attributable to the illness, serving simply as one of its more characteristic symptoms. From a narrative perspective, however, these accounts represent the person's active attempts to make sense of his or her experiences based on the fact that there is very little in the person's previous life that speaks directly to these concerns.[39]

Perhaps an example will help to illustrate the difference between these two points of view. In prior research,[24] we described the case of one young man with schizophrenia who attributed his difficulties to the effects of being poisoned by his parents. On the surface, this would appear to be a classic example of a delusion of the persecutory type. After getting to know this young man the following story emerged, which suggested that his conclusion was based on other factors in addition to his schizophrenia. He reported that he first experienced difficulties in high school with his memory, attention and concentration, and that this led to his grades dropping. Having been an 'A' student, and having never experienced anything like this before, he was at a loss as to what had gone wrong. The only explanation he could think of that would account for his intellectual deterioration was that he had brain damage, but he was not born with any birth defects nor had he had any traumatic brain injuries. He had not had such difficulties all of his life, and yet nor had they come on in an abrupt or sudden fashion. They had gradually built up incrementally over the previous few years but for what reason?

It must have been due, he reasoned, to an invisible yet toxic substance that had slowly been causing him brain damage. As it turned out, he had been exposed to just such a substance several days a week for the previous two years as he walked to and from his home to his part-time job at a tyre store. His route was along a busy interstate highway where cars and trucks were emitting exhaust containing carbon monoxide, a relatively invisible yet toxic substance. Walking along the edge of the interstate for the couple of miles it took him to get to and from work must have been the cause of his loss of cognitive capacity, mediated by effects of exposure to carbon monoxide on his brain. But where did his parents fit in? And how did he come to the conclusion that they had been poisoning him?

From his perspective, it was his parents' fault that he had to walk to and from work along the interstate highway, as they had refused to allow him use of one of their cars. As a result, when he was acutely upset, he blamed them directly for his exposure to the toxic substance that had caused his incremental brain damage. What suggests that this is more than just a delusional account is that the young man was relieved to learn that his condition was not due to irreparable brain damage but to schizophrenia, a disorder for which he could receive effective treatments and from which he could recover. As his cognitive functioning improved with treatment, his concern about possible brain damage was alleviated, and his anger at his parents dissipated.[24] As a result, what appeared to be his delusional ideation abated also, leaving him with a very different account of his last several years.

Adopting a narrative perspective in this way broadens our horizons concerning the range of factors that might influence a person's understanding of, and response to, the onset of a mental disorder. Working from such a position, Estroff and associates[40] referred to illness/identity work as the process by which a person learns about and incorporates psychiatric explanations once he or she comes into contact with mental healthcare or composes counterclaims about illness and self in reaction to a biomedical explanation. In their view, this process generates two main types of talk about self and illness: normalising talk, which disputes the assignation of illness and reauthorises either the condition as commonly occurring or the person as not sick, and illness identity statements, which include self-representations that incorporate illness.

Lysaker *et al*[41] emphasise the importance of removing obstacles from the person's capacity for dialogue between self-positions[13] to increase the complex, dynamic and diverse internal conversations of the narrator. In other words, people can entertain more than one perspective on their experience at any given time, and some people describe their silent deliberations between opposing perspectives as a useful way of adapting to the realities of having the illness.[42] Narrative can be a powerful means of stimulating and bringing to life such dialogue. In the same fashion, awareness of the barriers to forming such narratives and the effort to remove them and provide enabling conditions for their development can be crucial to recovery itself.

Building on the work of Estroff, Lysaker and others, we employed narrative constructs in the analysis of interview data in which people recovering from a psychotic episode described the experiences of self in relation to their illness.[35] Data for these studies were collected as part of the Yale Longitudinal Study[43,44] and included assessing participants who were hospitalised at one of Yale Medical School's four hospitals for a psychotic disorder. Assessments were conducted during hospitalisation, shortly after discharge, bimonthly for a year, and then every six months for an additional two years. Each assessment included the use of standard rating scales and an in-depth interview that was recorded and transcribed. Different qualitative analytic strategies were used and are described in greater detail in each of the studies themselves.[42,44]

In one of these studies[42] we identified five distinct categories that speak to different relationships that emerge in this process. In the first category, participants separated their 'healthy' self from their 'ill' self. This separation occurred at the narrative level, in the story the participant told and in which she created two subjects: 'myself' and 'myself when I am ill'. In the second category, contact replaced separation between the two selves. The healthy self remained a subject, whereas the illness became an object. In narrative terms, one can say that in this category, the 'healthy' self develops from focaliser to narrator, thus increasing his responsibility for his own personal story. In the third category, there was a transformation from a one-sided relationship in which the self tried to act on the illness, to a two-sided one in which the object (illness) was perceived as actively trying to influence the subject as well. At this stage, the more cohesive self was a more sophisticated narrator. The self used the narrator's position to change the object, the illness, making it more tolerable, which the narrator found to be empowering and which enhanced his or her capacity to cope. In the fourth category, the narrator had even more efficacy: she not only controlled the focus of the story, or the way in which it was told and made meaningful, but rather became the protagonist or her own story – that is, had control over the events and actions of the story itself and not only about the way it was told. In the fifth category, participants reached a point at which they demonstrated a capacity to integrate self and illness. They used the flexibility of narrative, incorporated with the dimension of time, to combine the different categories into a coherent whole. Thus, as seen above, allowing for multiple truths provides a foundation for the person to construct the narrative of his illness and himself in relation to it. This ongoing negotiation is important not only to separate the person's self from the illness, but also to construct a sense of self independent of the illness, as described in the following section.

The reconstruction of self through recovery narratives

Longitudinal studies conducted over the previous 30 years have demonstrated consistently that between 45% and 65% of people who meet established criteria for having a schizophrenic illness will experience significant, if not full, recovery over time.[7] Qualitative research conducted with this population suggests that an effective sense of self as a social agent and a restored life narrative are not only among the results of recovery, but also appear to play a crucial role in processes of recovery as well.[24] In this final section, we explore how this is so.

Among the more common disruptions reported by people with schizophrenia, in addition to threats to agency and identity, are experiences of decisions and actions being generated from somewhere outside of the person's own intentions,[45] a sense of the person no longer being rooted in history,[46] and a sense of being engulfed by the illness[47] and trapped in 'patienthood'.[48] According to Estroff,[49] this last disruption involves a social, as well as internal, process through which a once valued person is transformed into someone who is dysfunctional and devalued, first by others and then by himself as well. As she describes: 'a part time or periodically psychotic person can become a full time crazy person in identity and being.'[49] In this respect, she compares schizophrenia to other 'I am' illnesses in which the person's identity is taken hostage by the diagnosis, and hypothesises that the personal and social loss of self is actually one key component or even cause of chronicity.[49]

If these are the disruptions that the illness and its social impact introduce into the person's life, it stands to reason that processes of recovery will involve compensating for, if not altogether reversing, these effects. And this is, in fact, what we found in our earlier research involving follow-along, narrative inter-views with people recovering from schizophrenia. In our first study, for example, we described[44] a four-stage process of self and identity reconstruction involving the person: 1) discovering the possibility of a more active sense of self than that which had been taken over by the illness; 2) taking stock of the strengths and the weaknesses of this self and assessing possibilities for change; 3) putting into action some of the recently (re)discovered aspects of one's self and integrating the results of these actions into a revised sense of self; and 4) employing the enhanced sense of self to provide a refuge from the disorder, thereby creating additional resources for coping. What this research suggests is that instead of losing the capacity for narrative, people acutely or severely disabled by schizo-phrenia have seen their previous narrative diverted through a combination of internal and social factors to one confined largely to shame, passivity and helplessness. What is then required is a process through which this narrative can be salvaged by identifying and integrating the remaining aspects of self which have been preserved and/or unaffected by the illness.

This process can perhaps be captured well in a vignette that comes from a recent training course in which one of us was involved. In response to the trainer's description of several principles of recovery-oriented practice in mental health, a participant offered the Confucian proverb that, 'If you give a man a fish he will eat for a day, if you teach him to fish he will eat for a lifetime.' To this, another participant responded angrily: 'Yeah, that *sounds* great. But what if the person [with schizophrenia] doesn't have the capacity to learn to fish?!' After a short pause, a gentleman then stood up in the back row of the room, identifying himself as a person in recovery from schizophrenia. From his perspective, he offered: 'There are lots of other things to do besides fish.' In schizophrenia, it appears that recovery requires identifying those other things the person can still do in spite of the illness, gradually rebuilding a positive and effective sense of self based on the pleasures and satisfaction that come from exercising those aspects of self, and then using the enhanced sense of self which results as a resource in coping with, compensating for and overcoming those aspects of the illness which remain.[44]

Within the context of a condition as multidimensional and complex as schizo-phrenia, narrative is one of the few tools available that enable the person to weave back together a sense of who she is that both incorporates and yet extends beyond who she used to be prior to illness and who she has become due to illness. As we saw above, the emerging self may contain the changes and vicissi-tudes associated with living with the illness while simultaneously preserving a contradictory sense of the person's former life and projected future. While accepted discourse or reason would not be able to tolerate such opposing views existing side by side, narrative is flexible enough both to survive and to contain the apparent contradictions between self and illness. Even when appearing delu-sional to others, such narratives can serve as an organising mechanism for the person, offering the possibilities for control, continuity, flexibility and integration. What appears to be more important in characterising such narratives is not their content, but the opportunity they provide for the person with schizophrenia to regain ownership over his own story, and thereby his own life. In recovery nar-ratives what appears most important is that the person becomes the protagonist, the hero, of her own story, regardless of whether or not she learns how to fish or forgoes fishing in order to engage more effectively in other activities.

Conclusion

Life harbours an inherent tension between our universal, innate wish for completeness, coherence and continuity, on the one hand, and frequent confrontation with internal and external events that are experienced as fragmented, conflicting and discontinuous, on the other. Schizophrenia, along with the social and personal meanings it often holds and their many implications, poses a major challenge to any such desire for coherence and continuity. Without minimising the suffering unique to schizophrenia, it does share the characteristic common to traumatic events in that it generates a major interruption in the person's life story.[39] We have suggested, in contrast to the historical view of schizophrenia as a progressive disease, that this interruption does not constitute a permanent loss of self and narrative as much as a disruption from which the person can recover. To facilitate this process, we suggest focusing on the person's active efforts to regain and strengthen an effective sense of self and coherent life narrative rather than dwelling on the fact that these have been lost to the illness.

Imagine a computer virus suddenly randomly shuffling the thousands of words we composed here to convey our ideas. This disruption would pose a significant setback to our efforts to move ahead in developing, organising and sharing our thoughts on the topic. Although understandably annoyed, if writing this paper was really important and meaningful to us, at some point we would have no choice but to try to recall what it was that we were trying to convey and start writing again. There would be no short cut to the arduous task of gathering back together the scattered words into a new version of the chapter. Given that this is not a puzzle where each piece has its place, the resulting chapter would not and could not be the same. While we are not suggesting that the impact of a virus on a Word document is similar to the impact of schizophrenia on the life of a person, we offer this analogy to illustrate a point: life is constantly vulnerable to unwanted and unpredictable interruptions, and the effort to gather up the pieces and try to put them together again is one of the most important, adaptive, healing and creative processes of which humans are capable. Whether fixing the engine of a car, learning to play a new piece of music, or positioning personal belongings in a new house, the sanction to rearrange, put together, improvise, try again, negotiate and create meaning through the process is crucial. This is no less true in the case of recovery from schizophrenia.

Not only are people with schizophrenia entitled to make sense of their experiences, but this process is actually crucial to their ability to live with and recover from the disorder. The process of narrating suggests there is a narrator, an active agent, a self, authoring a new story. The process of authoring the story, in turn, helps to consolidate and integrate a sense of self. The interactive process we describe, and its role in recovery, suggest that mental health services should offer the opportunities and supports needed for people to be able to find, hold onto and reclaim their stories and their selves, and encourage them to use these as resources in overcoming and living beyond the illness.

Emphasising the importance of the person's self and narrative being at the centre of care is not obvious and nor should it be taken for granted. Traditional medical research and treatment have, in various forms and to various degrees, claimed ownership over definitions of illness and its treatment. While medicine appears to be shifting toward more consumer-directed care, we remain concerned that even this concept can be used to displace narrative. For instance, psychoeducational interventions focusing on insight and adherence might lose their effectiveness to the degree that they ignore, threaten or aim to replace the making of meaning and narrative processes.[50] No matter how improved new manuals may be, in that they provide useful information rather than theories that blame, and no matter how empowering they intend to be, by viewing patients as people who can learn about and understand their condition, they cannot simply replace one story – for example, bad mothers – with another prepackaged story which fails to speak to the person's own experiences, for example, a chemical imbalance. Scientific evidence is important, but only as one source of information and one thread in the person's tapestry; a tapestry that includes many other fabrics and hues. Within this larger and more complex picture, it is the narrating self and the construction of her ongoing story that must take, and remain, centre stage.

Acknowledgement

The authors wish to thank Drs Barbara Felton and Abraham Rudnick for their helpful comments on an earlier draft of this chapter.

References

1 Nassar S (2001) *A Beautiful Mind: the life of mathematical genius and Nobel laureate John Nash*. Simon & Schuster, New York.
2 Eigen M (1986) *The Psychotic Core*. Aronson, Northvale, NJ.
3 Laing RD (1978) *The Divided Self*. Penguin, New York.
4 American Psychiatric Association (1980) *Diagnostic and Statistical Manual of Mental Disorders* (3e). American Psychiatric Association, Washington DC.
5 Chaika E and Lambe RA (1989) Cohesion in schizophrenic narratives, revisited. *J Commun Disord*. **22**: 407–21.
6 Sass LA (1994) *Madness and Modernism*. Harvard University Press, Cambridge, MA.
7 Davidson L and McGlashan TH (1997) The varied outcomes of schizophrenia. *Can J Psychiatry*. **42**: 34–43.
8 Andreasen NC (1984) *The Broken Brain*. Harper & Row, New York.
9 Davidson L and Stayner D (1997) Loss, loneliness, and the desire for love: perspectives on the social lives of people with schizophrenia. *Psychiatr Rehabil J*. **20**: 3–12.
10 Morgan KD and David A (2004) Neurological studies of insight in patients with psychotic disorders. In: X Amador and A David (eds). *Insight and Psychosis*. Oxford University Press, New York.
11 Frank JD and Frank JB (1993) *Persuasion and Healing: a comparative study of psychotherapy* (3e). The Johns Hopkins University Press, Baltimore, MD.
12 Kleinman A (1988) *Rethinking Psychiatry: from cultural category to personal experience*. Free Press, New York.
13 Lysaker PH and Lysaker JT (2002) Narrative structure in psychosis. *Theory Psychol*. **12**: 207–20.
14 Leventhal H, Nerenz DR and Steele DF (1984) Illness representations and coping with health threats. In: A Baum and J Singer (eds). *A Handbook of Psychology and Health*. Erlbaum, Hillside, NJ.

15 Lobban F, Barrowclough C and Jones S (2003) A review of the role of illness models in severe mental illness. *Clin Psychol Rev.* **23**: 171–96.

16 Weinman J and Petrie KJ (1997) Illness perceptions: a new paradigm for psychosomatics? *J Psychosom Res.* **42**: 113–16.

17 Lobban F, Barrowclough C and Jones S (2004) The impact of beliefs about mental health problems and coping on outcome in schizophrenia. *Psychol Med.* **34**: 1165–76.

18 Freud S (2002) *The Wolfman and Other Cases* [translation Adey Huish L]. Penguin, London.

19 Edwards J and McGorry PD (2002) *Implementing Early Intervention in Psychosis.* Martin Dunitz, London.

20 Taylor SE, Kemeny ME, Reed GM *et al* (2000) Psychological resources, positive illusions, and health. *Am Psychol.* **55**: 99–109.

21 Kravetz S, Faust M and David M (2000) Accepting the mental illness label. *Psychiatr Rehabil J.* **23**: 324–32.

22 Moore O, Cassidy E, Carr A *et al* (1999) Unawareness of illness and its relationship with depression and self-deception in schizophrenia. *Eur Psychiatry.* **14**: 264–9.

23 O'Mahony PD (1982) Psychiatric patient denial of mental illness as a normal process. *Br J Med Psychol.* **55**: 109–18.

24 Davidson L (2003) *Living Outside Mental Illness: qualitative studies of recovery in schizophrenia.* New York University Press, New York.

25 Link BG, Cullen FT, Struening EL *et al* (1989) A modified labeling theory approach to mental disorders: an empirical assessment. *Am Sociol Rev.* **54**: 400–23.

26 Link BG, Cullen FT, Frank J *et al* (1987) The social rejection of former mental patients: understanding why labels matter. *Am J Sociol.* **92**: 1461–500.

27 Corrigan P, Watson AC, Heyrman ML *et al* (2005) Structural stigma in state legislation. *Psychiatr Serv.* **56**: 557–63.

28 Corrigan P, Watson AC, Gracia G *et al* (2005) Newspaper stories as measures of structural stigma. *Psychiatr Serv.* **56**: 551–6.

29 Torry EF (1983) *Surviving Schizophrenia: a family manual.* Harper & Row, New York.

30 Laroi F, Barr WB and Keefe RSE (2004) The neuropsychology of insight in psychiatric and neurological disorders. In: X Amador and A David (eds). *Insight and Psychosis.* Oxford University Press, New York.

31 Roe D and Kravetz S (2003) Different ways of being aware of a psychiatric disability: a multifunctional narrative approach to insight into mental disorder. *J Nerv Ment Dis.* **191**: 417–24.

32 Estroff S (2004) Subject/subjectivities in dispute: the poetics, politics, and performance of first-person narratives of people with schizophrenia. In: JH Jenkins and RG Barrett (eds). *Schizophrenia, Culture, and Subjectivity.* Cambridge University Press, USA.

33 Greenfeld D, Strauss JS, Bowers MB *et al* (1989) Insight and interpretation of illness in recovery from psychosis. *Schizophr Bull.* **15**: 245–52.

34 Roe D, Lereya J and Fennig S (2001) Comparing patients' and staff members' attitudes: does patients' competence to disagree mean they are not competent? *J Nerv Ment Dis.* **189**: 307–10.

35 Roe D, Weishut DJ, Jaglom M *et al* (2002) Patients' and staff members' attitudes about the rights of hospitalized psychiatric patients. *Psychiatr Serv.* **53**: 87–91.

36 Ridgway P (2001) Restoring psychiatric disability: learning from first person recovery narratives. *Psychiatr Rehabil J.* **24**: 335–43.

37 Jacobson N (2001) Experiencing recovery: a dimensional analysis of recovery narratives. *Psychiatr Rehabil J.* **24**: 248–54.

38 Davidson L, O'Connell M, Tondora J *et al* (2005) Recovery in serious mental illness: paradigm shift or shibboleth? In L Davidson, CM Harding and L Spaniol (eds). *Recovery from Severe Mental Illnesses: Research evidence and implications for practice.* Volumes 1 and 2. Center for Psychiatric Rehabilitation of Boston University, Boston, MA.

39 Davidson L (1993) Story telling and schizophrenia: using narrative structure in phenomenological research. *The Humanistic Psychologist*. **21**: 200–20.

40 Estroff SE, Lachicotte WS, Illingworth LC *et al* (1991) Everybody's got a little mental illness: accounts of illness and self among people with severe, persistent mental illness. *Med Anthropol Q*. **5**: 331–69.

41 Lysaker PH, Lancaster RS and Lysaker JT (2003) Narrative transformation as an outcome in the psychotherapy of schizophrenia. *Psychol Psychother*. **76**: 285–99.

42 Roe D and Ben-Yishai A (1999) Exploring the relationship between the person and the disorder among individuals hospitalized for psychosis. *Psychiatry*. **62**: 370–80.

43 Strauss JS, Hafez H, Lieberman P *et al* (1985) The course of psychiatric disorders III: longitudinal principles. *Am J Psychiatry*. **142**: 289–96.

44 Davidson L and Strauss JS (1992) Sense of self in recovery from severe mental illness. *Br J Med Psychol*. **65**: 131–45.

45 Carpenter WT Jr, Heinrichs DW and Wagman AM (1988) Deficit and non-deficit forms of schizophrenia: the concept. *Am J Psychiatry*. **145**: 578–83.

46 Kline J, Horn D and Patterson CM (1996) Meaning and development in the interpersonal treatment of severe psychopathology. *Bull Menninger Clin*. **60**: 314–30.

47 Lally SJ (1989) Does being here mean there is something wrong with me? *Schizophr Bull*. **15**: 253–65.

48 Roe D (2001) Progressing from 'patienthood' to 'personhood' across the multi-dimensional outcomes in schizophrenia and related disorders. *JNMD*. **189**: 691–9.

49 Estroff S (1989) Self, identity and subjective experiences of schizophrenia: in search of the subject. *Schizophr Bull*. **15**: 189–96.

50 Roe D and Yanos PT (2006) Moving beyond information and towards inspiration. *Behavioral Therapist*. **29**: 53–6.

Chapter 7

Motherhood versus patienthood: a conflict of identities

Janet Rhys Dent

In this chapter I discuss the memoir I wrote, a memoir about myself being ill. This is not the self-indulgent exercise it initially sounds: firstly, my memoir was written not just in an attempt to make sense of my experiences but also to connect with other women with life-threatening illness; secondly, this chapter is written to communicate the kind of conflicts of identity that illness provokes, and to reflect on the authorial construction of identities in an illness narrative. Autobiographical storytelling is drawn from 'multiple, disparate and discontinuous experiences and the multiple identities constructed from and constituting those experiences'.[1] Our identities are in a state of continuous flux in response to changing contexts over time and are framed by factors such as race, religion, ethnicity, education, sexuality, gender and class. It was my experience that sudden illness can suddenly interrupt these identities and throw them into confusion, inducing changes that are dramatic and intense. As Broyard wrote, 'My initial experience of illness was as a series of disconnected shocks, and my first instinct was to try to bring it under control by turning it into a narrative.'[2] In my own narrative I remember, reflect on and construct not only myself being ill but also the cultures that provoked or interacted with my responses to my illness. In this chapter I focus on the conflict between my identities as 'mother' and 'patient' and the way I constructed them in the act of writing. Thus, this analytical and interpretive chapter is a second step away from the immediacy of my original illness experiences but it is also another reflective step towards understanding their meaning. Before discussing four extracts from it, I explain the reasons why I chose to write my memoir and why I chose its particular form since both choices informed the way I constructed my fluctuating identities in the memoir.

The story of my illness explores many themes relating to myself, a woman patient, and the learning that took place during the acute phase of my hospital treatment. For example, there was the search for information about my illness that came to seem like an interactive relationship with my favourite internet search engine, nicknamed 'Gaia'; there was my membership of a support group, 'Bosom Buddies', as well as my passing obsession with self-help books and therapies; there was the time spent trying to make sense of the 'detour' in my illness in the form of my arm being accidentally paralysed during an operation; then there was the coming to terms with disfigurement, and, throughout all of this, the threat of premature death. Though all these themes relate to post-diagnosis, flitting around them are the various identities of my pre-illness life, trying to adapt to and often coming into conflict with my emergent role as 'patient', none more so than my identity as a mother.

I wrote my memoir of illness, just as other patients have done, to try to make sense of my experiences and to share them. It relates to the six months of my initial hospital treatment and takes the form of a story. This, many theorists believe, is the only conceivable form for a unified and purposeful telling of an individual life.[3–5] In the act of writing my story, I remembered facts and events, reflected on them, interpreted them, directed them and found meaning in them. By reading my story of the dilemmas, the vulnerabilities, and the sort of world in which a fellow patient finds herself, maybe my fellow women patients would enjoy reflecting on and comparing their own experiences of illness and above all, sensing the 'unity of human experience'.[6] I myself had read other women's illness memoirs, gaining comfort from stories like Meyer's in which she describes '…women like myself, the new citizens of this other country, a huge army of the wounded, each believing herself to be alone in her shock and grief';[7] and gaining political insight from accounts like Lorde's profound feminist analysis of her illness. In it she refers to 'the need for every woman to live a considered life': in doing so, we women become less willing 'to passively accept external and destructive controls over our lives and our identities'.[8] Another motive for writing my story was to attempt to capture the amazing breadth and richness of the world that I entered as a hospital patient and outpatient. I found myself in a world where the concept of what it was to live a 'good life' as a 'patient' gradually shed its passive connotations for me and took on a new meaning as active, dynamic and dialogical.

Each story of illness maps out a different territory of 'the considered life' and my own aim was to focus solely on that intense phase, the first six months of medical treatment. This is the period when so many ritualistic events occur such as testing, diagnosis, surgery and prognosis; the time when you are indisputably a patient; the time when you start to realise that for good or ill, life-threatening illness is not just a bodily event but a body-mind event that is throwing your old assumptions about yourself and the world into chaos; and it is the time you begin to glimpse new possibilities of connection with others and realise that this personal crisis is perhaps not such a personal one after all.

I had an idea what I wanted to say in my memoir and which approach to use but what to call the finished product? The audience I wanted to address was that of other women patients so it had to be a term that, as well as being accurate, had meaning and appeal for this diverse group and that was why I chose the term 'memoir'. There has been an explosion of memoirs in this age of self-disclosure, thus popularising both its aims and its form, and my methods fitted Barrington's description: 'Rather than simply telling a story from her life, the memoirist both tells the story and muses upon it, trying to unravel what it means in the light of her current knowledge.'[9] Barrington reflected the hopes I had for my reader, 'Your reader has to be willing to be both entertained by the story itself and interested in how you now, looking back on it, understand it.' Furthermore, the term 'memoir' would possibly indicate to readers that I would not be telling my complete life story but extracting a theme or themes from my life that would bind the work together.

It was only when I started looking at various forms of self-narrative that I realised the kind of memoir I was writing could be categorised as an 'autoethnography', a term that was first used in 1975 in an article by Karl Heider,[10] but did not gain wider currency until later. My memoir shares the characteristics of autoethnography (though there is no standard definition): autoethnography is an attempt to explain self to others; it attempts to see self as others might; it offers explanation of how one is 'othered'; it is about the writer as part of a group or culture; it attempts to explain differences from inside; it describes conflicts of cultures. My memoir is not always objective and sometimes my primary aim is to capture mood or feelings. Unlike many autoethnographies, my memoir is addressed specifically to the group that I am part of – other women patients. It fits Danahay's definition: 'autoethnography... can be done by an autobiographer who places the story of his or her life within a story of the social context in which it occurs.'[11]

The immediate impetus to write about my illness came from the taciturnity of the hospital medical staff. A few weeks after finishing surgical and radiotherapy treatment for breast cancer, I put in a request to look at my hospital medical notes. They duly arrived in the post in an A4 brown envelope. On reading them, I was disappointed by their minimalism and realised that I had hoped, naively enough, for a record that gave me some insight into my experience instead of just the bare recordings of injections, prescriptions and test results. It was then that I realised that I already had an idea of the sort of thing I had hoped to read, that I did not have to wait for doctors or nurses to interpret my illness for me and so I started to write my own account of my illness in a memoir that is now on its final draft with the working title, 'The Secret Life of a Woman Patient'. Its title refers to the sort of transformational experiences that underlie the bare and linear medical accounts of illness. Memories of illness can be unkind, recalling only the worst discomfort, the most humiliating moments and the darkest fears. What you remember may be just reflecting the habitual mood or outlook of your present self but inexorably you begin to turn these memories into the definitive 'factual' account of your illness. This was my experience until writing my illness memoir led me to remember and reflect on the joy and enlightenment that also formed my experience as a patient.

I found meaning in my illness and the meaning came from focusing on my memories and then portraying them in my writing through the various jumbled but pervasive identities that emerged as 'me', the narrator. Among these identities were 'patient', 'woman', 'writer', 'wife', 'Welsh', 'musician', and 'mother'. In this chapter, I mainly focus on my identities as 'mother' and 'patient', the transforming nature of the conflict between these two identities and the ways that I constructed them during my illness and in the writing about it. In particular I discuss them in relation to four extracts from my memoir.

Initially my entrenched concept of motherhood, based on the role of the all-powerful Welsh mother endemic to the village where I was brought up, conflicted with my emergent role as powerless patient and filled me with despair. Breast cancer is linked in so many ways with motherhood including semiotically, the breast, psychologically, the self-abnegating mother, and physically, the healthy, nurturant mother. These were the links that scared me when I was first diagnosed as a patient with breast cancer, making me feel that I was an inferior mother who was letting her children down. This fear permeates Excerpt 1.

This first excerpt is taken from near the beginning of the memoir when I begin to fear that illness might change my relationship with my three children, aged from 16 to early twenties. Having already discovered my breast lump and undergone initial tests, involving a mammogram, an ultrasound and a biopsy, I find myself rationalising my compulsion not to divulge any of this to the children.

Excerpt 1

I knew that I was a vital source of support to them [the children], the strong and selfless mother that they could rely on to be consistent however much their current lives changed. It would be foolish to worry them at this stage. It might all be for nothing. This waiting time was bad enough for me. Why inflict the worry on them? Why take away their faith in my health, in my strength, unless it was absolutely necessary? If it did turn out to be cancer, I would tell them then. I myself was still trying to make sense of what breast cancer meant. It was all a jumble in my mind waiting to be processed. If I myself found it confusing, how could I make a realistic and reassuring job of explaining it to the children?

...I was terrified by the prospect of facing up to my children's pain. I was scared not just for them but for me. I would find it painful to view their pain. My job was to protect them from pain not be the cause of it.

I was desperate to maintain my image of myself as a good mother. Since I was a little girl growing up in a tiny village in a South Wales valley, my ambition had always been the same.

When I was six a school inspector asked me, 'What do you want to be when you grow up?'

'A mother,' I said.

Being a friend of my father's, the inspector duly reported this back to him. Thus it entered the annals of family mythology, the perpetual feedback of my career destiny as a mother.

Now my power as a mother was threatened. Due to [my partner] Sam's career progression, we had moved house eight times since my son, my eldest child, was born and the frequent moves over the years had made the children and me a tight unit. I might now stop being the mainstay and driving force of my family's life, the archetypal strong Welsh mother role familiar to me since childhood might be lost. I might no longer be in control of family crises like exams, sports injuries or problems with girlfriends or boyfriends. My children might feel that they had to protect me rather than the other way around. How would I be able to deal with that? I would feel so sorry for them and guilty that I had let them down – I just could not imagine it. The best thing was to carry on as normal and not let them know anything about what was going on. Most likely, everything would turn out for the best and my results would clear me.

...After being diagnosed with breast cancer, I had no choice but to tell the children. I told them one by one but in such an upbeat way that they were left completely confused and unsure as to whether the diagnosis was anything to worry about or not. I was so horrified about using the word 'cancer', about myself to the children and having it intrude into my relationship with them that I completely minimised its significance.

The gist of what I said was, 'I've got breast cancer but it's not serious and I'll soon be better.'

> They went along with me and tried to appear unconcerned since that was how I obviously needed them to react. Left to try and work things out for themselves, they must have been aware of my evasiveness.
>
> Ceri [my daughter], was with me when Emma, a friend who had been diagnosed with breast cancer a year earlier, came round in the early evening bearing a massive bunch of pink roses and a card with the inscription, 'With love from one survivor to another.' I was touched by Emma's kindness but when I saw this inscription I froze. What if the children saw it? I immediately took the flowers into the kitchen to put them in a vase, and hid the card under the clutter in one of the kitchen drawers. The word 'survivor' implied that I was facing danger and it would frighten the children.

Here, early on in my story, is an ethical clash between my identity as a mother, which is based on a certain ideal of motherhood, and my new identity as a patient. A mother is the warm centre of the household, a rock, selfless, and at the same time magical and intuitive so that she knows what is best for her children. This was the ideal I had picked up from my mother, my grandmother, my aunts and my friends' mothers when I was a little girl. The Welsh 'mam', the stereotypical domestic matriarch, is part of Welsh culture. None of the mothers in our village had jobs for there was little work for women in that small valley. For most mothers, the chapel – the home of the stirring sermon, the Gymanfa Ganu (a festival of singing in four-part harmony), and the annual coach outing to the seaside – was their only non-domestic commitment. There, rich and warm though the culture was, patriarchy reigned. The minister was always male and the chapel elders who sat in 'The Big Seat' that undulated around the elite area immediately below the pulpit, were all men. Small wonder that the women claimed the domestic territory as their kingdoms and small wonder that I grew up associating those domestically devoted mothers with a strong kind of femininity and a selfless kind of power.

Now, in Excerpt 1, faced with serious illness, I 'know' that as an ill mother, I would be a failing mother. When breaking the news to the children, I am reluctant to voice the word 'cancer' with its clinging connotations of stigma and death, a symptom of 'the pervasive forms of cultural anxiety' identified by Stacey.[12] Cultural anxiety meets cultural anxiety, fear of illness meets fear of failure as a mother: my hope that 'my results would clear me', with its implication of a verdict of innocent or guilty is a recognition of my readily assumed role as the accused mother.

I refer in the excerpt to the frequent moves we as a family made because they had such a strong influence on my role as a mother. Because I was moving around from one place to another in England instead of living a rooted life in Wales, it became even more important to me to provide a stable childhood for my children, with myself as the centre and, in the absence of other stable influences, the mediator of their lives. It was the only way I knew to provide stability. Living in an alien country it was up to me to be not only their mother but also to compensate for the absence of the Welsh cultural influences of my own childhood. 'One's personal identity, insofar as it is tied to the interpretive appraisal of one's personal past as it takes place in autonarrative, is inseparable from normative ideas of what a life is, or is supposed to be, if it is lived well.'[13]

In Excerpt 1, my identity as a mother, formed by my rigid understanding what is a good mother, is flung into disarray by my new 'patient' identity with its connotations of weakness and uncertainty. My friend's phrase 'from one survivor to another' implies that the outcome of one's illness is self-determined, something I later find disturbing, and that it is a source of female bonding, something I later find to be true but at this stage its main effect is to frighten me because 'survival' is the antithesis of, and therefore implies the possibility of, death. So I 'tidy' the threat away 'under the clutter' in a kitchen drawer, hide it away from the children and me – another symptom of my evasiveness, a hopeless strategy to protect my children, control their experience and smother my own fears. This reaction is echoed in some respects by my mother's reaction to my news in Excerpt 2.

This passage relates to the week after I first discovered a lump in my breast, when I am still waiting for my diagnosis. From what I had read on various medical websites and from the ultrasound technician's comment, 'It's a hard lump,' along with the consultant's reaction, I suspect that the lump is malignant.

Excerpt 2

I told my mother. She said, 'Most breast lumps turn out to be nothing. Don't worry. You haven't got breast cancer. You can't have. You've never had very big, fleshy breasts.' Her voice rang determined and confident down the phone.

She cited the number of friends she knew whose breast lumps had turned out to be benign and, when I visited her in south Wales a few days later, she invited one of them, Gwyneth, a solicitor, over for a cup of tea after she had finished work. We sat in my mother's pink and cream sitting room, surrounded by family photographs including some of my late father. He had been headmaster of the town's comprehensive school and my brothers, Gwyneth and me had all been his pupils.

After a few minutes my mother said, looking at Gwyneth, 'Well, I'll leave you now while I go and make the tea. Gwyneth's going to tell you about her breast lumps.'

My mother turned to me. Still curvaceous and good looking with clear hazel eyes, surprisingly smooth skin and high cheekbones, she had maintained the fierce determination that I remembered from a childhood that was occasionally punctuated by long meal-time sieges: on such occasions we children would be allowed to leave the table only when we surrendered and force-fed ourselves nauseating tapioca pudding, prunes and custard, or some other hated food.

Now she said, 'Have a chat with Gwyneth.'

Gwyneth did not look at me but sighed and stretched her slim arms in the air so that the sleeves of her sleek grey suit fell into ripples around her elbows.

Gwyneth, my mother's loyal friend, normally full of chat about the latest events in her life, told me in a flat voice about the three occasions when her breast lumps turned out to be harmless cysts. Then she stared at her elegant narrow feet in their purple high-heeled shoes.

'Yes, but mine's a hard lump,' I said, explaining what I had learned about the geology of lumps.

Gwyneth shifted in her armchair as I spoke, and looked away from me at a photograph of my mother in smart suit and hat standing next to my father and surrounded by school governors after a school Speech Day

'But my lump might turn out to be nothing at all,' I conceded.

Gwyneth flopped back in her chair and smiled at me. 'Too true,' she said.

My mother returned. 'Gwyneth's told you, hasn't she,' she said and the subject was closed. My lump was a harmless cyst, just like Gwyneth's and it had been pretentious of me to think otherwise. I began to realise that my mother had a whole agenda of attitudes, including guilt that her daughter might have a serious disease, and disbelief that I, who unlike her was slim and small-breasted, could have such a seriously female disease as breast cancer. At the heart of her thinking was the thought that every mother has: that if anyone is going to have a serious illness, it should be the mother, not the child.

Though my mother is wielding power in a more overt way, her motives are the same as mine as revealed in Excerpt 1: fear, love, guilt and the determination to control events. There are also parallels in our attitudes to my authenticity as a breast cancer patient: my mother thinks that I am not female enough to have a 99% female disease like breast cancer that affects an appealingly female secondary sexual characteristic. Elsewhere in the narrative I admit that I find this aspect of the disease quite comforting: though I am losing part of a breast I am gaining validation as a woman, and hence as a mother. In this way I am allying myself, just like my mother, with 'a certain image of *'Woman'* that is the culturally dominant model for female identity'.[14] Yet, as is its wont, this dominant model is giving with one hand and taking away with the other – despite being the result of a female disease that is glamorised by the media, the mutilated breast is seen as a violation that discredits its owner's femininity.

I stayed with my mother for three days but these are the moments I chose to record in my memoir. I was engaged and threatened by them and I thought other women would relate to them in various ways or at least find them thought-provoking. It is likely that other significant moments occurred during those three days but they escaped my memory. Doris Lessing points out that, 'As you start to write at once the question begins to insist: Why do you remember this and not that? Why do you remember in every detail a whole week, more, of a long ago year, but then complete dark, a blank? *How do you know that what you remember is more important than what you don't?'*[15]

There were other events that I did remember but since they, in my consideration, did not relate to my story of illness, I omitted them. Selection is a vital part of writing a memoir and the criteria for the author are often those of relevance and of the value and interest to one's audience, not to mention the occasional failure of nerve arising from fear of exposure. However, had I written the events that I omitted, my story would be different. The flow of the story and the content of my next selection of material would be influenced by what I had already written. '…Narrators selectively engage their lived experiences through personal storytelling… [they are] in dialogue with the personal processes and archives of memory'.[1] Excerpt 2 is a fragment of memory that is now part of the complex construction that is the story of my illness.

Seeing the way my mother reacted to the challenge to her identity as a mother gave me an insight into the fragility of my own role and, paradoxically, it gave me my first glimpse into the freedom that comes with not clinging to a rigid ideal of motherhood. Smith and Watson's observation that 'identity as difference implies identity also as likeness' is also, of course, antithetically true.[1] The commonality of our identities as mothers and the kind of vulnerability revealed by my mother's response made me start to realise that control was also a part of my identity as a mother though not in an identical way. Comparing led to contrasting and, in turn, to questioning. What of mothers who did not seek this kind of control? I began to have the first intimations that change was possible and that there were many different ways to be a good mother.

Excerpt 3 records my thoughts as I enter hospital for a breast cancer operation.

Excerpt 3

Ward twelve, which was to be my home for the next five or so days, was housed in the same six storey block as the maternity unit. As I walked from the car park, I could see the window of the room where I had given birth to Ceri, 17 years ago. Fourth floor, second window from the left. The labour had been sudden and intense, too quick for a transfer to the delivery room as planned. After the birth was over, I was left alone, lying on a high trolley, with my tiny baby in a crib next to me. When she cried, instinct took over and I leaned down at a dangerous angle to scoop her up and breast feed her. Now one of the breasts that had nourished and comforted her had turned malignant. Seventeen years ago it had flowed with the vital proteins, minerals and vitamins of breast milk. Now it contained a dry, cancerous lump, full of malignant cells. The collision of the two locations, birth ward and breast excision ward, made me feel sentimental and self-pitying. Then I began to remember that this whole process had happened to millions of other women, including some of my closest friends, and there was never any reason why it should not happen to me.

This is also a passage about love and control. The central image is one of me selflessly rescuing my baby to feed her. I look back and reflect on the fact that where once I was an active, nurturing mother, now I am a passive patient, a body to be operated on. The body that is part of my identity as a mother is already changed by the tumour and will be further altered by the operation to come when a part of my breast will be cut out. Patienthood will steal a bodily sign of my identity as a mother. The mother–patient conflict has become dramatic and it is not surprising that there is an element of self-dramatisation in the above passage. Sentimentality, grandiosity and other enjoyable indulgences can creep in to even the most low-key autobiographical accounts. Here, I am viewing and portraying myself as something of a heroine. Whilst ambivalent about including this excerpt in my memoir, I left it in because it is a true reflection of how I felt when I was writing it and of my thoughts as I entered hospital. There is a circularity to it.

I state that I was self-pitying and then write that final sentence that shows me pitying myself, as victim mother and victim patient, even as I write about my self-pity. As Broyard writes, 'Illness is primarily a drama, and it should be possible to enjoy it as well as suffer it.'[2]

Illness was to force my children and me into different roles, loosening our hold on our traditional family roles of earth mother, child son, and child daughters. My first intimations of this come immediately after my operation.

Excerpt 4

...sure enough, back in the ward, with the help of the morphine I had been administered, I became more cheerful. Lewis, my son, was the last of the family to visit, having jogged the ten miles across the park and streets that lay between his apartment and the hospital. He loomed over me to kiss me. Then, hot and larger than life, he flung himself into the black plastic arm-chair, his sweat glossing the matt black vinyl. His health and energy filled the room so that he seemed to have come from a different planet. Yet, as we talked in that alien room, cast in the unfamiliar roles of visitor and bed-ridden patient, I felt a new kind of communication and intimacy between us that was not just drug induced.

This was a pivotal moment, what Bruner refers to as a 'turning point.' The image of Lewis looming above me is the counterpoint to the image in Excerpt 3 where I loomed over my passive newborn baby. It is I who am now lying prone, help-less and dependent. I am no longer the 'strong' one thereby putting the children into the 'weak' role. From this moment in the hospital room implicit in my rela-tionship with the children, grew the acknowledgement that I was weak and strong just like them, just like everyone else. Turning points, says Bruner, 'repre-sent a way in which people free themselves in their self-consciousness from their history' and are 'steps towards narratorial consciousness'.[16] Extracts 1–3 reveal the persistent challenges that illness makes to my identity as mother but it is only in this one that I have intimations that my role as mother is changing. Bruner observes that it is unsurprising that turning points occur at moments when the culture gives more freedom. In the above excerpt, illness has given me the free-dom to abandon my habituated mother role. The room seems 'alien', my son seems to have come from 'another planet'. I am in a different world and am free to act in a different way. The hospital environment constrains me but it also releases me. Trapped in hospital, I am free to slough off at least part of the con-strictive skin of all-powerful motherhood. This freedom from my own conception of motherhood, as well as what I believed to be others' expectations of me as a mother, gives me the chance to recognise the nuances of a new kind of commu-nication and a new kind of identity. However, it is not just 'freedom'. The free-dom comes in parallel with a surrender. I had loved being a 'Welsh mother'. It had been my ambition since I was a little girl, since even before I had confided in that school inspector, and there was a delight and exhilaration in the role and its raw femininity and power. Alas, illness had highlighted its weaknesses and writ-ing about it helped me to recognise and hence accept, at least partially, its loss.

Out of hospital and unable to use my right arm, literally 'disarmed', I grew accustomed to being waited on by my children, from cups of coffee to meals to chauffeured journeys. It was a physical confirmation of the shift in our relationships, which grew freer and deeper. It did not happen all at once or even completely, for my original construct of being a 'good' mother is still part of me but in time I learned to relax into the new order and in time I realised the rigidity of my previous concept of motherhood.

Writing my story and reconstructing myself in that story, not only led me to reassess my past: I began to realise I was being reshaped by a new regime, that of my illness and its treatment. I myself was living in and writing this regime even as I became aware of it. This is what Hertz defines as being reflexive: 'it is to have an ongoing conversation about experience while simultaneously living in the moment.'[17] I also began to reflexively recognise that I, my 'self', had already been moulded by other regimes like the traditional, domestically all-powerful Welsh 'mam' whose cultural examples, not least those of my own mother and grandmother, surrounded me when I was growing up. By challenging roles such as this one, illness gave me an indication of the deeper experience of life and the deeper connection with others that living in a more enfranchised way can bring. My writing was having the kind of effect that Henry Miller observed, '[Writing] lifts the sufferer out of his obsessions and frees him for the rhythm and movement of life by joining him to the great universal stream in which we all have our being.'[18]

I became conscious of my identities as intersectional. I was not only Welsh and a mother, I was a Welsh mother. I was not only a woman and a patient but a woman patient whose idea of patienthood had been initially determined by the way busy medical staff viewed the steady flow of breast cancer patients as anonymous bodies. These and other identities ebbed and flowed, merged and conflicted. Writing about them revived my sense of self in many diverse ways, reminding me of the joy of 'going with the flow' and the futility of struggling to fit an inauthentic identity.

It was cathartic to become aware that my experience as a patient was not simply the depressing, simple, linear affair of my pre-writing memory. Yet, just as there is no fixed self so there is not one unified story. My memoir is not the real story but just one of the real stories, just as this chapter is but one of the real stories. There is no fixed story, no fixed self because we are never 'fixed': we are always in action, 'being' in time and circumstance, and the reflexive process is part of this state of being. Even now there is a part of me that holds that pre-memoir account as the truth even as I remember the complexities, the joys and the sorrows of the fluctuating identities and the true and transformative experiences I present in my memoir. It is all the truth and it is all my 'self'. Writing my memoir helped me to recognise this.

References

1 Smith S and Watson J (2001) *Reading Autobiography*. University of Minnesota Press, Minneapolis.
2 Broyard A (1992) *Intoxicated By My Illness*. Fawcett Columbine, New York.
3 Brady H (2003) *Stories of Sickness*. Oxford University Press, Oxford.
4 Frank AW (1995) *The Wounded Storyteller*. University of Chicago Press, Chicago.
5 McAdams DP (1993) *The Stories We Live By*. The Guildford Press, New York.

6 Lopate, P (1997) *The Art of the Personal Essay: an anthology from the classical era to the present.* Anchor, London.

7 Meyer M (1993) *Examining Myself.* Faber & Faber, Winchester, MA.

8 Lorde A (1996) The Cancer Journals. In: A Lorde (ed) *The Audre Lorde Compendium.* Pandora, London.

9 Barrington J (1997) *Writing the Memoir: From Truth to Art.* Eighth Mountain Press, Portland, Oregon.

10 Heider KG (1975) What Do People Do? Dani Auto-Ethnography. *Journal of Anthropological Research.* **31**: 3–17.

11 Reed-Danahay DE (ed) (1997) *Auto/Ethnography.* Berg, London.

12 Stacey J (1997) *Teratologies: a cultural study of cancer.* Routledge, London.

13 Freeman M and Brockmeier J (2001) Narrative integrity. In: J Brockmeier and D Carbaugh (eds). *Narrative and Identity.* John Benjamins, Amsterdam/Philadelphia.

14 Braidotti R (1986) Nomadic subjects: embodiment and sexual difference in contemporary feminist theory. In: M Eagleton (ed). *Feminist Literary Theory.* Blackwell Publishers, Oxford.

15 Lessing D (1995) *Under My Skin: Volume One of my Autobiography, to 1949.* Flamingo Rpt, London.

16 Bruner J (2001) Self-making and world-making. In: J Brockmeier and D Carbaugh (eds). *Narrative and Identity.* John Benjamins, Amsterdam/Philadelphia.

17 Hertz R (ed) (1997) *Reflexivity & Voice.* Sage Publications, California.

18 Miller H (1992) *Stories, Essays, Travel Sketches.* MJF Books, New York.

Chapter 8

Becoming a nurse: 'It's just who I am'

Don Flaming

As a nurse educator, I am always interested in exploring a nursing student's experience of becoming a nurse. Other people agree and have used sociological concepts – for example, professional socialisation and role socialisation – to explore nursing students quantitatively.[1–6] Researchers approach the topic qualitatively too, using phenomenology,[7–10] grounded theory,[11] and ethnography.[12] These authors all provide insights into the nursing student experience, but theirs is not an explicitly ontological orientation. In a research project in which I asked student nurses to explore with me their experience of becoming a nurse, I was guided by an ontological theory, not a sociological or psychological one. I am not an expert in ontology, but I believe that philosophical insights into experiences are valuable for nursing practice and nursing education, just as I value insights from sociology or psychology. The purpose of this paper is not to present a comprehensive report describing a research study, but by referring to my study, I will argue that Ricoeur's narrative theory as reflected in *mimesis* and his ontological theory, when used together, is a fecund approach for researching constructions of self identity.

Because my primary purpose is *not* to provide a comprehensive description of a research report, I do not give a full account of my research project, but I will provide a brief description of the context. After receiving approval from an ethics review board, I obtained consent from 10 senior level female nursing students who all had a previous degree in another non-nursing discipline. I would not necessarily have excluded men from the sample, but none volunteered. I interviewed all volunteers in this convenience sample at least once and interviewed four of the more reflective and articulate students two more times. I interviewed students over three academic semesters and a professional transcriptionist transcribed these 18 interviews. I have not included excerpts from all 10 women in this chapter, even though all participants contributed to my understanding, because my primary purpose is to highlight the appropriateness of Ricoeur's thought in research, rather than presenting a typical research report.

As a nurse researcher, I am most familiar with other nurse researchers who have transposed Ricoeur's philosophical thinking to the research process. Nurses have studied a variety of experiences, including suicidal psychiatric patients;[13] the experience of caring for a person acting in a disturbing manner;[14] the meaning of fatigue in women with fibromyalgia and healthy women;[15] the suffering experienced when being cared for;[16] understanding a woman's experience of an acute myocardial infarction;[17] patients' experience of understanding stroke;[18] the experience of being a hospice nurse;[19] living with symptoms related to Parkinson's disease,[20] and exploring registered nurses' meaning of identity.[21] All these researchers reference Ricoeur's[22] *Interpretation Theory: discourse and the surplus of meaning* as the main source for their understanding of interpretation.

Based on Ricoeur's book, these researchers incorporate a three-stage process in their interpretive process and move from understanding (a naive grasping of the story) to explanation (structural analysis of the text) to comprehension (referred to by the authors as a more sophisticated mode of understanding). I suggest that this three-step approach, while useful, is insufficient to grasp Ricoeur's understanding of interpretation. Some researchers do reference Ricoeur's[23] collection of essays called *From Text to Action* when describing their interpretive approach, but an exploration of his methodology – that is, *mimesis*, not just the method he describes – helps me better understand the interpretive experience. None of the above researchers reference *Time and Narrative*,[24] the book in which Ricoeur discusses *mimesis*, the cornerstone of his interpretive theory, though as the title suggests, Ricoeur believed that temporality is key to understanding how people construct narratives of the self.

By combining Ricoeur's well known narrative theory as a research methodology and his ontological theory as a guiding framework for research, researchers are presented with a fecund combination that can result in a decidedly philosophical exploration – that is, ontological, of the experience under consideration, rather than, for example, a sociological or psychological understanding. I was informed by a Ricoeurean interpretive research methodology and Ricoeurean ontology when studying nursing students' developing self identities as nurses. Some people might assume that 'self identity' is a psychological concept and in many contexts it is, but Ricoeur uses the word philosophically, that is, from an ontological perspective when exploring how people understand themselves as a particular human being. Ricoeur states that his book, *Oneself as Another*,[25] is a comprehensive exploration of his ontology and, to my knowledge, Fredriksson and Eriksson[26] are the only other nurse researchers who – in their study focusing on the ethical foundations for a caring conversation – reference this book.

When I asked a participant in my study, Kate, why nursing suited her, she said: 'It's just who I am.' From Kate's perspective, the practice called 'nursing' fits her self identity – that is, her ontology, just as nursing fits Anne, another participant. Anne believes that the fit between her self and nursing practice is 'even becoming stronger. When I was applying for the programme, no one would have told me it's a calling…but now that I'm in it, it does.' Being *called* to the nursing profession is more than just having the necessary educational credentials or having the necessary skills, it is rather a feeling of fulfilment at a deeply personal level; being called means being fulfilled ontologically. No conflict exists between what Anne does in her nursing practice and what her self, developed over time, does as a human being. She says: 'I don't have to act the role of nurse… It's too difficult to be different [than being myself]… It just feels right. That was a sign to me.' Anne would deceive herself and others if she acted differently when nursing than when she is not nursing. Being a different person in one situation to the next would not only be difficult, but would also be quite wrong because she would be lying to herself.

Ricoeur's understanding of narrative and *mimesis*

For Ricoeur, a person's personal narrative is a construction that helps that person make sense of who she or he is as a human being. This construction is a temporal one because people include past, present, and future action in these narratives.

Actions are meaningful because they reflect who that person is as a particular human being. When fully explored, these actions are actually public expressions of inward motivations. Action reflects a person's ontology and, 'To identify an agent and to recognize this agent's motives are complementary operations.'[24] By exploring motivations for action, not from a psychological perspective, but from an ontological one, we learn who that person is as a particular human being. Valdés characterises Ricoeur's interpretive process as 'the return to the world of action as the basis for all meaning; this is the cornerstone of Ricoeur's theory of interpretation'.[27] Ricoeur, a philosopher, never describes a research method, but his methodology is especially appropriate for my study because when asked about becoming a nurse, participants reflected on their actions with other people. By doing this, students made sense of, or constructed, who they are and who they want to be as a nurse.

Ricoeur believes that temporality is part of a person's narrative construction. Self-understanding cannot occur by considering our personal experiences chronologically; rather, Ricoeur assumes that certain experiences in a person's life are more important than other experiences when constructing a comprehensible self. He states that the self is an empty place if, indeed, each experience in our lives is given equal importance. Our self is vastly richer if time is considered to be 'a gathering moment where expectation, memory and present experience coincide'.[28] From a Ricoeurean perspective, participants in my study offer a richer understanding of their selves becoming nurses when, through the narrative, they gather together their past, present and future experiences. These nursing students remember, and anticipate, important events that shape who they are as nurses or who they will become as nurses. Their memory of past experiences, their experience of the present, and their imagined future experiences coalesce into a constructed self identity – a particular human being. Participants state categorically that the experiences they consider when thinking about becoming a nurse are not limited to nursing education, but include many life experiences which play an important role in their construction of self.

Ricoeur's unique contribution to interpretive theory, according to Pranger,[29] is his understanding of *mimesis*. This concept, from the ancient Greeks and the classical theory of art,[30] describes how people imitate past experiences so that others can experience the event. This imitation often occurs through artistic means, including narratives, and unlike narrativists before him, Ricoeur describes three subsets of *mimesis*.[24] He does not suggest a linear process, but by separating *mimesis* into three parts, he can clarify the holistic nature of the interpretive process. The subsets are *mimesis*$_1$ (prefiguration or prefigured time), *mimesis*$_2$ (configuration or configured time), and *mimesis*$_3$ (refiguration or refigured time). They are 'a fundamentally circular and reflexive nature of understanding'.[31]

Mimesis$_1$

Mimesis$_1$ refers to preunderstandings of the world that motivate a person to act. For Ricoeur, *mimesis*$_1$ 'applies to our existing common sense view of the world in which we have gained experience of organizing events in a particular way in making sense of the world'.[32] The phrase 'common sense' implies that people act on the basis of their understanding of shared assumptions about the world. Some assumptions are explicit – for example, linguistic rules shared by a group so that communication can occur – but some (or perhaps many) prefigurations are powerful, yet remain implicit and even inarticulable. *Mimesis*$_1$ is 'prefigured time' because many of our assumptions are not consciously figured into narratives of the self. Exploring these hidden assumptions can provide ontological insights into motivations to act as a particular human being.

Mimesis$_1$ is so important in the interpretive circle that Ricoeur states: 'The most fundamental condition of the hermeneutic circle lies in the structure of preunderstanding which relates all explication to the understanding which precedes and supports it.'[33] For researchers, exploring preunderstandings gives glimpses into the motivations behind a particular person's actions. While Britzman does not use the word *mimesis* in her study exploring the experience of students studying to be teachers, she states that student teachers 'bring to teacher education their educational biography and some well worn and commonsensical images of the teacher's work'.[34] These biographies and 'commonsensical' images are, I think, examples of the prefigurations (*mimesis*$_1$) that Ricoeur discusses.

Mimesis$_2$

Ricoeur refers to *mimesis*$_2$ as *emplotment* or the 'configuring time' that, using an analogy of place, lies between the prefigured time reflected in *mimesis*$_1$ and a person's interpretation of a narrative reflected in *mimesis*$_3$. Configuration 'opens the kingdom of *as if* [italics in the original]'.[24] *As if* does not mean that a person's narrative is fiction, in the sense of having no basis in real events; rather, when people construct narratives, they really believe that events happened just as they remembered them. Their narratives are fiction in the sense that a person's prefigurations, both implicit and explicit, taint the narratives. Narratives of the present are never innocent; they are always guilty of being influenced by the past and future. People impose an order on their experiences, or construct their experience, as they try to imitate their actual life experiences in memories for themselves and for others.

Using an aural metaphor, Ricoeur[35] states that an isolated experience in a person's life is mute by itself and is made 'eloquent' only when that experience is placed in a meaningful relationship with other events in life through narration. Only through this emplotment does time become configured human time as an expression of self identity, not simply as events occurring in a chronological order. I assume that participants' stories about becoming a nurse are not exact reproductions of their life events, but that a particular participant, shaped by her own prefigurations, uses a particular construction to make her experience comprehensible.

Mimesis$_3$

Mimesis$_3$ is *refigured* time and refers to 'the time of action'[24] when the text meets, and inevitably influences, the reader. The text refigures the reader's life because, Ricoeur assumes, reading a text always has an impact upon the reader. In fact, for Ricoeur, the entire interpretive process (*mimesis*) is worthwhile only because narratives produce a reader to act. Ricoeur states that: 'At the end of our investigation, it seems that reading is the concrete act in which the destiny of the text is fulfilled.'[24] In interpretive research, the 'concrete act' happens when the researcher reads the transcribed interviews. The researcher realises that the *mimetic* arc (or what some writers refer to as the *mimetic* circle) is complete in *mimesis*$_3$ because a researcher's interpretation of participants' narratives is grounded in that researcher's own prefigurations (*mimesis*$_1$). The relationship between *mimesis*$_1$ and *mimesis*$_3$ is so close that when we, as researchers, interpret our participants' narratives, we are also interpreting our own self. The interpreter becomes the interpreted as our own prefigurations shape our interpretation of someone else's narrative. When talking or writing about their research, interpretive researchers construct their own emplotments of participants' emplotments. When engaging in this construction, researchers must consider how their own prefigurations affect their decisions. This personal vigilance should not paralyse a researcher, but should remind us that no one 'real' construction of the self exists. While similarities in researchers' constructions may very well exist if several people analyse the same data, researchers' selves, who are different from each other, will inevitably construct different interpretations of participants' selves. Through engagement in this study, for example, I found important prefigurations that included memories of my mother as a nurse, of experiences of my own nursing education, and of the curricular theory that I read.

Like any text, participants' words, once spoken, have a 'semantic autonomy'[22] allowing me, or forcing me, as a researcher reading transcripts to interpret them. Because a text is distanced from the original speaker (nursing student) – an 'exteriorization of discourse'[22] – I have the opportunity to think about the implicit and explicit meanings of participants' narratives. As a researcher, I want to always privilege participants' narratives, but reading their texts is to 'conjoin a new discourse [mine] to the discourse of the text [participants' words]'; interpretation is 'the concrete outcome of conjunction and renewal'.[23] Even if I remain acutely aware of my own assumptions and try to limit their effect on my decisions, my interpretation of participants' stories is inevitably influenced by my own discourse that joins the discourse of participants. I construct my own meanings of the meanings that participants have constructed. Through this process, 'the text's career escapes the finite horizon lived by its author. What the text says now matters more than what the author meant to say'[22] because the way I interpret the text motivates me to think and act in a certain way, even if that was not the author's intent.

This *distanciation* is an integral part of Ricoeur's theory because 'each text is free to enter into relation with other texts'.[33] The text 'no longer coincides with what the author wanted to say, verbal significance and mental significance have distinct destinies'.[36] Not only is the text distant from the author, but the text is also distant from the original situation and audience, thus allowing for – or necessitating – even more interpretive freedom. A reader of any text, and that includes researchers who read transcripts of participants' interviews, *reconfigure* these texts to meet their own *configurative* needs. Once written, a text becomes autonomous, but, as I said earlier, researchers cannot simply put words into the mouths of participants to meet the researchers' needs. When researchers write their interpretation of participants' experiences, the written work is nestled within a constant tension between a participant's constructed meanings and the researcher's own constructions of those constructed meanings. An individual researcher's written work about a phenomenon reflects the way that the researcher chooses to re-present participants' experiences.

Tantillo describes this important characteristic of narrative work by stating that interpreters 'read the text semantically as a work of meaning that is disconnected from the [original] author's subjective, mental intention'.[37] Usher, referring to interpretive and hermeneutic research, describes a 'double hermeneutic…because both the subject (the researcher) and the object (other people) of research have the same characteristic of being interpreters or sense seekers'.[38] Participants in my study interpret, or make sense of, their experience *as if* their experience were shaping their becoming a nurse. My own prefigurations bias me as I interpret or make sense of their interpretations *as if* my interpretations make sense to me. You, the reader of my interpretations of participants' interpretation, are even further removed from the participants' narratives because, just as I reconfigure participants' texts when writing this chapter, you reconfigure my words *as if* they make sense to you.

Ricoeur's ontology or self identity

Ricoeur's ontological theory of personal identity fits well with his narrative theory. In *Oneself as Another*, he specifically explores how people develop a self identity, for example, we all have names that provide some stability for our self identity. I am Don ever since I was born and I will continue to be Don until I die and even thereafter in people's memory. During my life, however, I have changed and will continue to change physically, mentally, emotionally and spiritually. I am a very different individual now from when I was born, yet I am still Don. Relating this to my research study, participants enter nursing education with a self identity, but their experience working with patients, with other students, with other nurses, and with other healthcare professionals, somehow changes who they are or changes their self identity. Ricoeur's work helps me understand why participants say, on the one hand, that nursing education does not change them, yet also say that nursing practice does change them.

Ricoeur addresses this philosophical impasse regarding continuity of identity and change – (Is a ship that has all of its parts replaced over time the same ship now as when it first sailed? After an organ transplant, is the recipient the same person?) – by distinguishing between *idem*-identity and *ipse*-identity. The former type of identity is the stable, unchanging sense of identity required for a person to feel grounded as a particular human being. If, however, a person is too grounded or too sedimented in the past, then that person cannot deal philosophically with the changes that a self inevitably experiences. An understanding of identity as *ipse*-identity, on the other hand, allows people to easily accept that stability and change are not mutually exclusive. A person's self identity as selfhood (*ipse*-identity) allows for change without the threat of that person becoming completely unidentifiable. Using a metaphor of place, and using classic examples from philosophy, Ricoeur suggests that an individual's narrative of self sits somewhere between the extreme of (a) the Cartesian *cogito* that traditionally reflects a static, immutable, exalted and cognitively objective self ('I think, therefore, I am'), and (b) a self that is completely shattered or dispersed, as Nietzsche suggests when he writes, 'God is dead'. In a philosophical way, Ricoeur promotes the idea that a healthy self identity happens when someone constructs a self based on a foundation that does not change so much that all former identity is lost, all the while being aware that a self does change somewhat so that all experiences can be incorporated into a coherent self.

Dunne thinks that Ricoeur advocates a self that is best explored through narratives and goes 'beyond sovereignty [*cogito*] and deconstruction [Nietzsche]'.[39] By interpreting an individual's narrative, we can explore *who* someone is (or is becoming). Because a person needs to have some grounding – that is, their *idem*-identity, a self is not, as a Nietzschean might say, merely a 'linguistic or rhetorical flourish'.[40] Diane Fuss,[41] a feminist thinker, agrees that when we think about our identity, we cannot delete all notions of self (although she believes that we do need to problematise them), lest we become an undifferentiated mass. To deconstruct identity, as she advocates, is not the same as disavowing identity, and I think this is Ricoeur's point, too. The 'nominal essence' or 'strategic essentialism' described by Fuss reflects the fact that we have some stability, even as we also experience change.

Relating the distinction between *idem*- and *ipse*-identity to nursing students becoming nurses, students reflect the Cartesian *idem*-identity when they deny that nursing education changes them in any way. Yet, they also describe changes to their self, not just increased knowledge, but at the level of *being* an excellent nurse. Jill, for example, talks about changing a core understanding of social rules. Early in her nursing education, as part of the morning routine, a nurse asked her to check a patient's vital signs and Jill had to become someone different from who she usually was:

> Sometimes you ignore your social conscious. This one time I was supposed to be doing a vitals check. The patient was sleeping. I came back out… In normal life, someone is sleeping, I am not going to go wake them up and piss them off!

I can relate to Jill because I clearly remember the first time I had to take the morning vital signs. Because I, too, was following the social rule that sleeping people are not to be disturbed (a prefiguration or *mimesis*₁), I stood in the hallway by the closed door for several minutes, unsure of what do to. I finally entered the room timidly, but I then wondered whether I should open the blinds, or whether to turn the lights on, or attempt to take vital signs in the very dim lighting. Both Jill and I had to change our prefigurations and change our assumptions about relating with other human beings.

A temporal understanding of a participant's personal ontology

Ricoeur's thinking helped me frame participants' constructions of self as being temporal understandings because their past life experiences and their anticipated experiences as nurses strongly influence their present understanding of becoming a nurse. Nursing education, participants say, does not alter their basic sense of self, and never will, but experiences with patients mean that they express themselves through *nursing* actions, something they have not done before. Paula, for example, believes that she can express her pre-existing commitment to compassion when providing nursing care. Being compassionate is an integral part of her self identity and she cannot imagine *being* without being compassionate. Her compassion did not suddenly develop in nursing education, but she brings this already existing self to nursing; she offers her compassion to nursing. The only difference now is that she has different opportunities to express her compassion. Compassion is 'the core of all the things that I do' and always being compassionate is integral to her self identity as Paula.

Engaging in nursing practice fits Kate's personal ontology too, because her experiences in nursing education are congruent with her experiences as a human being. She uses an image of Velcro to describe the close fit between her own self and nursing. Nursing, she says, 'came and attached itself [to me]…like Velcro'. Just as Velcro needs two complementary pieces that fit snugly together to create a strong bond, Kate believes that she bonds strongly with nursing. A conversation she had with a grade 8 teacher is a good example of her constructed, temporal understanding of self:

> I had this really amazing teacher in eighth grade, Mr Bowen, and I remember coming to him and saying, 'I understand everything we're learning in this class, but I just can't seem to get these straight As, like all these other kids in the class, who I know don't understand it as well, but they get these amazing marks. And he said to me, 'Oh, you know Kate, they're a bunch of sold-by-the-side-of-the-road long stemmed roses and you're a wild flower and you'll come into your own and when you do everything will make sense and you don't have to worry about all these other people.' And he was so right! And I want to write him a letter now that I'm here and I feel that so deeply. Because I feel like in my evaluations from my clinical instructors and some of my professors and some of the things I read in my paper, I feel like they see me as I see me, maybe, and that has never happened before in university, or in glimpses. I think that's the biggest confirmation of why I'm supposed to be a nurse, want to be a nurse.

By becoming a nurse, she has opened up like a flower to her true self. In fact, she feels obliged to become a nurse: 'I'm supposed to be a nurse.' Rather than this obligation being a burden, however, she understands it as being a positive development in her life. She is 'able to express the elements of myself that are unique', which, until now, being in nursing education, have been muted.

Anne states that nursing is 'better suited for my person'. By judging what suits her as a person, she has a sense of self identity. Part of that identity is working with people, rather than working with inanimate objects. Recently, she had a job working with objects and felt too much stress because she needed to work with people. She did not become a people person until after entering nursing school and she assumes that she will always be a people person. Because nurses work closely with people, becoming a nurse is congruent with Anne's constructed self identity. Another participant, Lisa, also needs an ontological fit between her work and her 'real me'. She left a career in the sciences in order to 'live a happy life' because she can now work with people. Her perspective reflects a temporal understanding of self because she compares her past unhappy life experiences with her current happy ones in nursing education.

Ricoeur uses the word *character* in his ontological theory, but researchers rarely, if ever, use that word in their research. I suggest that exploring character as a philosophical concept when engaging in research can help us understand the nursing student experience. *Character* comes from the Latin and means 'to scratch, to engrave',[42] suggesting that someone's character is a relatively permanent mark of who that person is as a particular human being. Anne states that contemporary nursing education remains silent about students' character, but that educators should not ignore this important aspect of being human:

> *[University education]* is all about consumerism. We pay money to get an education. You guys have a product. We buy that product. We are like a sausage factory, I think, because of money. We are, unfortunately. Things like character, or addressing character, that component we were talking about, it gets shuffled to the side because we need to learn how to do an injection or we need to do this… Maybe we will come back to that and realise that we can't ignore things like character.

Character has been important in nursing's past when, for example, educators admitted only students with good character. Rafferty writes about the politics of nursing knowledge and states that the first official nurses in the mid-Victorian era were 'defined in terms of character rather than intellect. A good nurse could not be turned out from bad material'.[43] Nursing education was a 'moral process, involving the development of character and self control rather than "mere" academic training'.[43]

For all participants in this study, good nursing practice is more than competently applying a skill set, but includes being a certain type of person. Some described this more explicitly than others, but all agreed that exhibiting certain personal characteristics or being a certain kind of self – having a certain character – is essential for good nursing practice. As Anne states:

> We know it's *[nursing]* not just tasks. It's so much more and it's really how we are as people. So we need to reflect. We need to examine ourselves and need to have other people challenge us in that capacity… It makes you a better person for sure.

Ricoeur uses *character* when describing the continuity of self that people experience over time, even as they inevitably change: 'Character…designates the set of lasting dispositions by which a person is recognised.'[25] A person's action when exploring character is paramount because, as stated earlier, a person's dispositions or character are understood or made manifest by that person's actions. A person's habitual ways of acting distinguish that person from another person. We talk about a person acting 'out of character' when their actions surprise us. Dunne[44] reflects the emphasis on action, too, when exploring character and states that while people can understand theory without action, they cannot understand character without action. Participants state that nursing was the 'right fit' for them and I interpret this to reflect Ricoeur's understanding of character. Their nursing practice (or nursing action) reflects their own usual or habitual patterns of thinking and acting. Paula reflects the importance of appropriate character for nurses when she states that, after providing care for someone, she wants that person to walk 'away not thinking about the care [they received]. They walk away thinking about the whole of me.' She wants patients to remember *who* she is as a whole person – her character, her disposition – more than remembering completed tasks.

For Anne, strong personal prefigurations (*mimesis*$_1$) include a strict, Catholic upbringing and a father who insisted that she always be a 'proper girl'. In her family, one way to be proper was to respect others, especially those people who are in vulnerable situations. Because she just assumes respect is important in being human, she habitually (or characteristically) respects others. This prefiguration from Anne's childhood reflects what MacIntyre calls 'standards of excellence'[45] that guide members of any community and become 'scratched' or 'engraved' on them. Individuals in a particular community measure their own actions against these standards, either explicitly or implicitly, as a way to distinguish themselves as a member of that community. Ricoeur refers to MacIntyre too, and states that people compare their own actions in relation to the 'ideals of perfection shared by a given community of practitioners and internalised by the masters and virtuosi of the practice considered'.[25] For Anne, members of her community – for example, the Roman Catholic church, her family – respect vulnerable people and this expectation from her past shapes Anne's own character or her own habitual way of acting, a good example of the temporality of self-narratives.

Participants talk about life experiences in their own character development. To develop good character, people need to practise good character through relevant experiences. Experience as a good teacher, however, is not just being exposed 'to 'one damned thing after another' but rather of particulars giving rise to, and then being perceived in the light of, universals'.[44] Remembering past actions and their consequences helps a person consider specific actions in current and future situations. Considering these past specific actions and outcomes results in better judgements and actions the next time a person faces a similar situation. Interestingly, several participants wonder how younger students without many life experiences can provide appropriate care. Tracy (aged 26) states: 'I would be scared of nursing at 18… I can't imagine being 18 in nursing at all.' She now sees how important her life experiences are when she is making patient care decisions. Life experience helped build an important ontological foundation for her current nursing practice. She now has a firm footing that she perceives younger students do not have. When thinking about students just out of high school, she remembers what she was like at that age and cannot imagine that young students can provide appropriate nursing care. Tracy's incredulity can only occur with a temporal understanding of becoming a nurse. She remembers the kind of person she was eight years ago and states: 'So, having eight years of life just teaches you a lot of things that you don't necessarily know where they come from, but they're there.'

Two suggestions: exploring health/illness experiences and implications for educators

I have two suggestions that incorporate the arguments I present in this chapter. First, Ricoeur offers an appropriate framework methodologically and philosophically when studying any experience related to health and illness. Researchers, for example, could explore the experience of someone becoming a person with diabetes or becoming a person with chronic lung or heart disease. They could also study a person's ontological experience of cancer remission or gaining increased mobility after joint replacements. Research studies do exist that explore patient experiences with these diseases and illnesses, but few researchers have used an explicitly ontological framework as a guide for an empirical study.

My second suggestion relates to the education of health professionals. I assume that many readers of this chapter are, like me, involved in educating health professionals. In a recent editorial,[46] Tanner wonders whether nurse educators should also explore students' selves (or their ontology), rather than assuming that an improved curriculum will automatically improve graduates. Rather than just wondering about an individual student's ontology, I think educators should explore that student's temporal understanding of their self identity. Doing so would help educators understand what motivates a particular student to a particular action. Since completing this project, I pay more attention to a particular student's prefigurations about their nursing practice and my own refigurations of that practice. By pressing students to articulate assumptions about their nursing actions, that is, by asking them to seriously consider their ontological motivation to act, I have had some success in helping students understand how their actions affect patient care. I take students to a psychiatric unit and two students' nursing practice improved when we worked together to articulate some negative prefigurations they had about patients with psychiatric conditions. By reflecting on their deeply held assumptions, that is, *mimesis*₁, both of them told me how much they had grown, not only as nursing students acquiring more knowledge, but also as human beings who will inevitably interact with mentally ill people outside of nursing. They had reconstructed their self identity, or who they were at an ontological level, and that resulted in more appropriate nursing actions. Through self-reflection, they identified certain characteristics, or dispositions, that they wanted to change to become better nurses. They had come to nursing with some prefigurations that, upon reflection, limited their effectiveness and they were willing to change their self in order to improve their care for patients.

In conclusion, in any research project, the underlying methodological framework and any framework guiding analysis should be compatible. Because Ricoeur offers both a methodological perspective through *mimesis* and a framework for thinking about participants' experiences from a philosophical perspective, his thinking is especially appropriate for my own study, as well as for researchers exploring many phenomena that involve human beings.

References

1 Clayton GM, Broome ME and Ellis LA (1989) Relationship between a preceptorship experience and role socialisation of graduate nurses. *J Nurs Ed*. **28**: 72–5.
2 Colucciello ML (1990) Socialisation into nursing: a developmental approach. *Nursing Connections*. **3**: 17–27.
3 Coudret NA, Fuchs PL, Roberts CS *et al* (1994) Role socialisation of graduating student nurses: impact of a nursing practicum on professional role conception. *J Prof Nurs*. **10**: 342–9.
4 Du Toit D (1995) A sociological analysis of the extent and influence of professional socialisation on the development of a nursing identity among nursing students at two universities in Brisbane, Australia. *J Adv Nurs*. **21**: 164–71.
5 Itano JK, Warren JJ and Ishida DN (1987) A comparison of role conceptions and role deprivation of baccalaureate students in nursing participating in a preceptorship or a traditional clinical program. *J Nurs Ed*. **26**: 69–73.
6 Nesler MS, Hanner MB, Melburg V *et al* (2001) Professional socialisation of baccalaureate nursing students: can students in distance nursing programs become socialized? *J Nurs Ed*. **40**: 293–302.
7 Diekelmann N (1993) Behavioural pedagogy: a Heideggerian hermeneutical analysis of the lived experience of students and teachers in baccalaureate education. *J Nurs Ed*. **32**: 245–50.

8 Diekelmann N (2001) Narrative pedagogy: Heideggerian hermeneutical analysis of lived experiences of students, teachers, and clinicians. *Adv Nurs Sci*. **23**: 53–71.

9 Kosowski JM (1995) Clinical learning experiences and professional nurse caring: a critical phenomenological study of female baccalaureate nursing students. *J Nurs Ed*. **34**: 235–42.

10 Fagerberg I and Ekman S (1998) Swedish nursing students' transition into nursing during education. *Wes J Nurs Res*. **20**: 602–20.

11 Gregg MF and Magilvy JK (2001) Professional identity of Japanese nurses: bonding into nursing. *Nurs Hlth Sci*. **3**: 47–55.

12 Holland K (1999) A journey to becoming: the student nurse in transition. *J Adv Nurs*. **29**: 229–37.

13 Talseth A-G, Lindseth A, Jacobsson L *et al* (1999) The meaning of suicidal psychiatric inpatients' experiences of being cared for by mental health nurses. *J Adv Nurs*. **29**: 1034–41.

14 Hellzen O, Asplund K, Sandman P-O *et al* (1999) Unwillingness to be violated: carers' experiences of caring for a person acting in a disturbing manner. An interview study. *J Clin Nurs*. **8**: 653–62.

15 Söderberg S, Lundman B and Norberg A (2002) The meaning of fatigue and tiredness as narrated by women with fibromyalgia and healthy women. *J Clin Nurs*. **11**: 247–55.

16 Sundin K, Axelsson K, Jansson L *et al* (2000) Suffering from care as expressed in the narratives of former patients in somatic wards. *Scand J Car Sci*. **14**: 16–22.

17 Svedlund M, Danielson E and Norberg A (2001) Women's narratives during the acute phase of their myocardial infarction. *J Adv Nurs*. **35**: 197–205.

18 Nilsson I, Jansson L and Norberg A (1997) To meet with a stroke: patients' experiences and aspects seen through a screen of crises. *J Adv Nurs*. **25**: 953–63.

19 Rasmussen BH, Sandman P-O and Norberg A (1997) Stories of being a hospice nurse: a journey towards finding one's footing. *Canc Nurs*. **20**: 330–41.

20 Caap-Ahlgren M, Lannerheim L and Dehlin O (2002) Older Swedish women's experiences of living with symptoms related to Parkinson's disease. *J Adv Nurs*. **39**: 87–95.

21 Fagerberg I and Kihlgren M (2001) Experiencing a nurse identity: the meaning of identity to Swedish registered nurses two years after graduation. *J Adv Nurs*. **34**: 137–45.

22 Ricoeur P (1976) *Interpretation Theory: discourse and the surplus of meaning*. The Texas Christian University Press, Fort Worth, TX.

23 Ricoeur P (1991) *From Text to Action: essays in hermeneutics II*. Northwestern University Press, Evanston, IL.

24 Ricoeur P (1984) *Time and Narrative (vol 1)*. University of Chicago Press, Chicago, IL.

25 Ricoeur P (1992) *Oneself as Another*. University of Chicago Press, Chicago, IL.

26 Fredriksson L and Eriksson K (2003) The ethics of caring conversation. *Nurs Ethics*. **10**: 138–48.

27 Valdés MJ (1991) Introduction: Paul Ricoeur's poststructuralist hermeneutics. *Ricoeur Reader: reflection and imagination*. University of Toronto Press, Toronto.

28 Reagan CE (1996) *Paul Ricoeur: his life and his work*. University of Chicago Press, Chicago, IL.

29 Pranger MB (2001) Time and narrative in Augustine's *Confessions*. *J Religion*. **81**: 377–93.

30 Gadamer H-J (1997) *Truth and Method* (2e, rev). Continuum, New York.

31 Fisher L (1997) Mediation, *muthos*, and the hermeneutic circle in Ricoeur's narrative theory. In: M Joy (ed). *Paul Ricoeur and Narrative*. University of Calgary Press, Calgary.

32 Brown T and Roberts L (2000) Memories are made of this: temporality and practitioner research. *Br Ed Res J*. **26**: 649–59.

33 Ricoeur P (1981) *Hermeneutics and Human Sciences*. Cambridge University Press, Cambridge.

34 Britzman DP (1991) *Practice Makes Practice*. State University of New York Press, New York.

35 Ricoeur P (1991) The human experience of time and narrative. In: MJ Valdés (ed). *A Ricoeur Reader: reflection and imagination*. University of Toronto Press, Toronto.

36 Ricoeur P (1973) The hermeneutical function of distanciation. *Phil Today*. **17**: 129–41.

37 Tantillo M (1994) Ricoeurean hermeneutics: its application in developing a contextual understanding of human experience. In: P Chinn (ed). *Advances in Methods of Inquiry for Nursing*. Aspen Press, Gaithersburg, MD.

38 Usher R (1996) A critique of the neglected epistemological assumptions of educational research. In: D Scott and R Usher (eds). *Understanding Educational Research*. Routledge, New York.

39 Dunne J (1996) Beyond sovereignty and deconstruction. In: R Kearney (ed). *Paul Ricoeur: the hermeneutics of action*. Sage, London.

40 Van den Hengel J (1994) Paul Ricoeur's *Oneself as Another* and practical theology. *Theol Stud*. **55**: 458–80.

41 Fuss D (1989) *Essentially Speaking*. Routledge, New York.

42 Woolfe HB (ed) (1976) *Webster's New Collegiate Dictionary*. Thomas Allen & Son, Toronto.

43 Rafferty AM (1996) *The Politics of Nursing Knowledge*. Routledge, London.

44 Dunne J (1997) *Back to the Rough Ground*. University of Notre Dame Press, Notre Dame, IN.

45 MacIntyre A (1984) *After Virtue* (2e). University of Notre Dame Press, Notre Dame, IN.

46 Tanner C (2004) The meaning of curriculum: content to be covered or stories to be heard? *J Nurs Ed*. **43**: 3–4.

Chapter 9

They stole my baby's soul: narratives of embodiment and loss

Alastair V Campbell and Michaela Willis

This chapter is written from the perspective of the retained organs controversy, which was uncovered by the Bristol and Alder Hey inquiries and investigations.[1,2] One of us (Michaela) suffered the double trauma of the death of a baby and retention of his heart, without her knowledge or consent. Michaela also chaired the Bristol Heart Action Group, which campaigned successfully for an inquiry at Bristol, and she was appointed as a member of the Retained Organs Commission. The other (Alastair) was appointed vice-chair of the commission. A year earlier, Alastair had suffered the loss of a daughter, who died of cancer at the age of 36. At his daughter's request, an autopsy was performed. (She wanted to have the efficacy of the complementary therapy she had used tested.) Her organs were not retained after the autopsy. For the authors, as for most other members of the commission, the powerful emotions generated by this controversy were an unforgettable experience. Commission meetings were held in public, and on several occasions the anger and grief of affected families interrupted proceedings or brought them to a halt. Pathologists were described as 'butchers', comparisons were made with the holocaust, and the commission members themselves were accused of a cover-up and of complicity in professional wrongdoing.

This chapter seeks to explore the roots of this powerful reaction to the widespread practice of retaining organs and tissue without the knowledge and consent of relatives. We suggest that we see here two different narratives, the professional story and the family story, narratives so different that the narrators simply talk past each other. The inquiries revealed unbridgeable differences in understanding between the professionals and the bereaved families. This showed a failure of communication, beneath which, we suggest, lay the dualistic approach of scientific medicine, with its treatment of the body as an object of study. The lay (non-medical) view of the body is quite different from the medical one. In the lay view bodies are seen as integral to persons, though also often distinguished from them – for example, when the person no longer seems present after a major brain injury – 'It doesn't seem like him any more.' Even when the person seems to have 'left the body', however, the mortal remains form a powerful reminder of the person once intimately known. For this reason, the unconsented removal of parts of a dead body is seen as an attack on a lost loved one and as an affront to the feelings of those who mourn the dead. We shall argue below that a richer understanding – one which acknowledges the significance of such 'embodied selves' in peoples' stories of their lives and in the lives of those they love – will serve medicine much more adequately than over-rationalistic accounts, which see the body as merely a container for consciousness.

Two narratives in non-communication

In *Doctors' Stories*, Kathryn Hunter describes what she calls the 'narrative incommensurability' of doctors' and patients' accounts of illness:

> The patient's account of illness and the medical version of that account are fundamentally, irreducibly different narratives, and this difference is essential to the work of medical care. Sick people who seek a physician's advice and help are in quest of exactly this difference, for physicians are believed not only to know more about the body but also to see its disorders clearly and without shame. Yet because it is scarcely acknowledged by either patient or physician, the difference between their accounts of the patient's malady can warp understanding between them.[3]

As we see from this quotation, Hunter is not deploring the fact that the narratives are incommensurable – she sees this as necessary if medicine is to offer help to the patient. Things go wrong, however, when the difference between the narratives is not acknowledged and understood, and this wrong is compounded, when, as in the retained organs controversy, the medical narrative persists past the point where it is either necessary or useful.

Let us compare, then, the way relatives saw the retention of organs after postmortem examination with how it was conceptualised by some of the professional bodies, who gave evidence to the Chief Medical Officer's (CMO) Summit on Organ Retention. The evidence of relatives is fully available from the documentation of the summit and also from the two inquiry reports of Bristol and Alder Hey. We can give only a few brief excerpts to convey the profound feelings experienced by so many families:

> To take all Stephen's organs from his body and store them for ten years without establishing a definitive cause of death is unacceptable. His parents buried him ten years ago as a shell. It is like grave robbing before being put in the grave. His body had been mutilated.[2]

> You relive the moment that she died over and over again. I have flashbacks of what they have done and what you imagine they have done. I had a dream the other day that I said to someone in the hospital where I work 'what is in the cupboard'. When we opened it there were three jars: one with babies' hearts, one with babies' lungs and one which looked like peas. When I looked closer they were eyes... I have a great big empty void inside.[2]

> ...they were devastated to hear that their daughter's tongue had been retained, and the father protested silently outside Alder Hey... They describe the hospital as having stolen their daughter's body, which was white as driven snow. It was reduced to skin and bone by predators and it must never happen again.[2]

> She is emotional for several reasons. The first is the deceit involved. She did not know what had happened to her daughter or that she had been desecrated. Alexandra had been stripped bare of everything and somebody believed they had the right to do it and to return her apparently complete for funeral purposes but in fact without her

internal organs. For five years she believed Alexandra was intact and at rest.[2]

> The worst aspect, I mean, it is an awful trauma having Bethan operated on. The one thing as a father one enjoys is having a sense of control over your son's life, but then with the operation, you lose that control, but then to further lose that control after death in this way is so upsetting.[1]

Compare this testimony from relatives with some of the written evidence given by professional medical associations to the CMO's summit:

> The fact that in the past many families have not been informed in detail about what a postmortem examination entails...invariably reflected a simple and understandable wish to spare them further anguish and distress at the time of bereavement.[4]

> The Royal College of Surgeons deprecates the retention of organs and tissues following postmortem examinations or surgical operations without appropriate informed consent having been given.

> The college believes that sensible measures should be introduced to allow for the continuance of retention of organs and tissues for scientific research and for teaching purposes.[4]

> It must be recognised that the retention of organs and tissues has been common practice, world wide, for centuries, and has formed an essential part of medical education and research, both undergraduate and postgraduate. The frequency of autopsy has declined over the past two decades to the detriment of education, and further obstacles to the use of autopsy are to be deplored.

> It is also regrettable that there have been implications that such storage of organs and tissues has been thoughtless, cavalier or macabre.[4]

> It is perhaps a paradox that in an age when we have more understanding than ever before of the nature of human life and the biology of the human body, we are more distressed than at any time in human history about what is perceived as inappropriate disposal of the whole human body or part of it... This is a philosophical puzzle...[4]

Perhaps this last quotation is the most powerful indication of the narrative dissonance of the medical and lay understandings of the body. The president of the Royal College of Paediatrics and Child Health cannot understand how, with such improved knowledge of the *biology* of the body, relatives can feel distressed when they discover that they have buried a body 'stripped of organs'. We see similar bewilderment among the physicians and surgeons, to whom the most important thing is the medical progress made possible by organ retention. The pathologists worry that the good intentions of the past (not to cause distress) will be overlooked. This is the medical story: it simply creates a different world from that of the grieving and angry relatives.

Such a clash of narratives is not restricted to the medical world. The philosopher, John Harris, shows similar puzzlement and disapproval, when considering the controversy over organ retention and the proposals for a more respectful treatment of human remains:

> A quite absurd, if understandable, preoccupation with reverence and respect for bodily tissue has come to dominate discussions of retained tissues and organs in the wake of the Alder Hey revelations. We do not normally feel this reverence for our bodily remains, tissue and organs when alive – why suddenly this morbid *postmortem* preoccupation?[5]

Harris's disrespect for respect in this situation stems from his commitment to a valuation of human life in terms of identity based on consciousness. He shares this with the philosopher John Locke, who gave an account of human identity based solely on awareness and memory. Such a view leaves no room for the significance of the body, though it lends itself well to the scientific paradigm on which medical practice is usually based. (One of us, Alastair, has explored this problem with John Harris's view of the body at greater length in a chapter in a forthcoming book entitled *Why the body matters: reflections on John Harris's account of organ procurement.*[6])

Embodiment, vulnerability, and loss

It would be naive to suppose that these two discourses can easily be reconciled. Indeed there is no need to do so, provided we understand that they serve different purposes. The medical discourse is functional for achieving the goals of scientific medicine, in which the body as object is required in order to create the generalisations that allow for differential diagnosis and (some kinds of) therapeutic intervention. Even in the realm of the living, however, it is now well recognised that such distancing and objectifying of the body has detrimental effects on health, and offers only limited scope for effective recovery from illness.

When medicine extends uncritically into the realm of the dead and supposes that 'this malformed and damaged heart' (to be stored in a jar for further study) is the same as 'my child's heart' (soon to be buried with my child's body), then it loses the plot completely. But, due to the god-like status that society has accorded doctors, the scientific account of the body becomes the only 'rational' one. The meanings attributed to the parts of the body by doctors and by the lay public are in reality completely different, and each has its own rationality. Intimate relationships never concern merely a meeting of minds or of Lockean self-valuing pools of consciousness! The physical body of the person loved is fully part of the love that parent feels for child or wife for husband. This embodiment of the person does not suddenly disappear in death, though, of course, it soon becomes necessary to let go of the body and live only with the memory and mental images of the person now dead. A mother cuddling her dead child, a husband kissing the cold brow of his wife's dead body, are not acts which *deny* the death of the person. They are part of the story of human lives shared and of the pain which comes from parting.

For these reasons, we believe that the narrative that best explains why unconsented organ retention was such an affront is one that focuses on embodiment of the self. In speaking of 'embodiment' we refer not just to issues concerned with respect for the dead, but also with the way in which we experience ourselves, other selves and the world around us. These experiences of embodiment are characterised by closeness, vulnerability and loss.

Emotions, the body, and the narrative self

At this point in our discussion some lines from a poem of Philip Larkin's come to mind:

> I would not dare
> Console you if I could. What can be said,
> Except that suffering is exact, but where
> Desire takes charge, readings will grow erratic?[7]

The striking contrast between the philosophical and medical narratives about the treatment of the bodies of the dead and the lay narratives of the same events stems from the centrality of emotion in personal relationships. In the retained organs controversy, families were criticised for letting their feelings run away with them, and it was suggested that the media were deliberately manipulating emotions to get a good story, with headlines such as 'They stole my baby's soul'. According to *The Times*, this outpouring of emotion badly damaged medicine:

> The body parts furore triggered an irrational and emotional backlash against pathology and organ donation, the effects of which are still being felt. A recent survey published in *New Scientist* found that one in ten pathology posts is vacant, as doctors shy away from joining a profession so widely caricatured as ghoulish.[8]

So now the families, traumatised by the deception and concealment of the organs controversy, must bear the blame for the problems of pathology! This moral condemnation is echoed in John Harris's description of opposition to the use of organs as 'wicked'.[9] Clearly, emotions can blind our better judgement at times and some powerful emotional reactions can have their own momentum, in which the wholeness of the self is engulfed and our identity lost. But without emotion we are no selves at all. We become distanced from our body and unable to create personal relationships or respond to the lives of others. It is as much the continuity of emotion as the continuity of memory and consciousness that gives us that unique phenomenon we call personal identity.

The neurophysiologist, Antonio Damasio, in a work criticising the influence of the mind/body dualism of Descartes on modern medicine, has written powerfully about how it is emotion that gives us our distinctive identity as humans:

> At first glance there is nothing distinctively human about emotions, since it is clear that so many non-human creatures have emotions in abundance; and yet there is something quite distinctive about the way in which emotions have become connected to the complex ideas, values, principles and judgments that only humans can have, and in that connection lies our legitimate sense that human emotion is special. Human emotion is not just about sexual pleasures or the fear of snakes. It is also about the horror of witnessing suffering and about the satisfaction of seeing justice served; about delight at the sensuous smile of Jeanne Moreau or the thick beauty of words and ideas in Shakespeare's verse; about the world weary voice of Dietrich Fischer-Dieskau singing Bach's *Ich habe genug*…[10]

So, reading again the narratives of the affected relatives, we can see how it is the emotional loading of the memory that makes it distinctively and painfully theirs: the dreadful images of the body as an empty shell; of the horrifying cupboard full of specimens that once were hearts or eyes of living babies; the depredation of a daughter's white body; the anger at the removal of a dead child's tongue; and the sense of loss of control when you can do nothing to protect your own child. These are all the responses of people in close human relationships.

It is pointless to suggest that these narratives of anger, grief, and loss are one-sided or irrational. They are what they are: the living memory of emotional trauma, which will be forever part of the identity of those experiencing them. There is no 'real' or 'better' or 'more rational' self, floating above the emotions of our daily bodily lives. There is only the lived self and there is only the one narrative of our bodily experiences, a narrative that is ours alone.

Conclusion: Embodiment and medicine

So what might this all mean for the practice of medicine? At one level, the retained organs controversy has brought to the fore some much needed changes in medical practice. New legislation should ensure that the removal and use of organs without consent cannot happen again. The powerful reaction of relatives to the discovery of retention has also brought about changes in medical practice, with a better understanding of how to help people facing the trauma of bereavement. But at a deeper level there is probably still a long way to go before medicine can rediscover the lost dimension of embodiment. This entails seeing the strength, but also the limitation, of the 'scientific' approach to medical practice. It requires the ability to respond to the emotional and not merely the physical aspects of people's lives.

A good place to start will be in the training and practice of doctors themselves, enabling them to reflect on their own embodiment. Medical training is beginning to respond to the demand that it produce doctors with a richer understanding of the whole person in medicine. For example, Jaye[11] reports on the responses of general practitioners who were introduced to the concept of embodiment as part of a postgraduate course in medical anthropology. One of the most interesting responses came from a practitioner who realised that medical training and practice had distanced her from her own body, to the extent that she failed to recognise even her own need for medical care:

> There wasn't time to think, there wasn't time to…be compassionate, you didn't have time to get to know people, you were running to physically keep up… I knew I had asthma, but I didn't realise that's what was doing it and I couldn't understand why I felt exhausted all the time… I felt numb, I did feel distanced from my own body… I think you become less human. And you didn't expect to see yourself as human.[11]

These telling words illustrate how the objectification of the patient's body, which scientific medicine encourages, can affect the practitioner's *own* bodily life to an almost lethal extent. Allowing the medical narrative to include an awareness of the doctor's own bodily reactions might indeed transform medical practice. It could be a meeting place for the medical and lay narratives at those times in medical practice when what the patient or family needs is a humane understanding of a shared vulnerability. We need to recover the wisdom of the old adage: physician, heal thyself.

References

1 Bristol Royal Infirmary Inquiry (2000) *Interim Report of the Bristol Royal Infirmary Inquiry.* Central Office of Information, London.
2 Royal Liverpool Children's Inquiry (2001) *Report of the Royal Liverpool Children's Inquiry.* Stationery Office, London.
3 Hunter KM (1991) *Doctors' Stories: the narrative structure of medical knowledge.* Princeton University Press, Princeton.
4 Chief Medical Officer's Summit on Organ Retention (2001) *Evidence Documentation.* Department of Health, London.
5 Harris J (2002) Law and regulation of retained organs: the ethical issues. *Leg Stud.* **22**: 527–49.
6 Campbell AV. Why the body matters: reflections on John Harris's account of organ procurement. In: S Holm, M Hayry and T Takala (eds). *Life of Value.* Amsterdam and Rodopi, New York (in press).
7 Larkin P (1988) *Deceptions, Collected Poems.* The Marvell Press, London.
8 *The Times* 6 December 2003.
9 Harris J (2003) Organ procurement: dead interests, living needs. *J Med Ethics.* **29**: 130–4.
10 Damasio A (2000) *The Feeling of What Happens.* Vintage, London.
11 Jaye C (2004) Talking around embodiment: the views of GPs following participation in medical anthropology courses. *J Med Ethics: Medical Humanities.* **30**: 41–8.

Index